HEART RATE VARIBILITY ESSENTIALS

DISCOVER HOW YOUR HABITS SHAPE THIS VITAL BIOMARKER

BY ANN PATRICK

Copyright © 2024 by Ann Patrick

All rights reserved.

No portion of this book may be reproduced in any form without written permission from the publisher or author, except as permitted by U.S. copyright law.

Contents

Introduction	1
1. Decoding HRV: The Basics and Importance	6
2. Practical Insights into HRV Monitoring	13
3. Habits & Factors that Influence HRV	22
Stress	23
Diet	26
Physical Activity	29
Sleep Quality	32
Hydration	35
Age	38
Genetics	41
Medical Conditions	44
Inflammation	48
Medications	51
Body Weight	54
Smoking and Alcohol Consumption	57

Environmental Factors	61
Breathing Patterns	65
Social Interactions	69
Mindfulness and Meditation	73
Time of Day	77
Caffeine and Stimulants	81
Nutrient Deficiencies	85
Posture	90
Marijuana	95
4. Creating Your HRV Improvement Plan	100
Conclusion	105
References	107

Introduction

Welcome to *Heart Rate Variability Essentials: Discover How Your Habits Shape This Vital Biomarker*. If you're here, you're not just committed to taking your health and fitness to the next level. You're ready to take the reins of your well-being. You're someone who understands that small, informed changes in your daily habits can lead to significant improvements in your overall health. This book is designed with you in mind—health-conscious individuals, fitness enthusiasts, and anyone eager to harness the power of Heart Rate Variability (HRV) to optimize their health strategies. It's not just about learning; it's about empowering yourself to make the right choices for your health.

Why I Wrote This Book

Hi, I'm Ann Patrick, and I'm thrilled to share my journey with you. My profound interest in health and fitness led me to delve into various biomarkers, and HRV emerged as a game-changer—an often overlooked yet incredibly powerful tool. Over the years, I've experienced firsthand how understanding and monitoring HRV can revolutionize our health, training, and recovery approach. This book is a testament to my passion and drive to provide clear, actionable advice.

What You'll Learn

This book is more than just a theoretical exploration of HRV. It's a practical guide that will equip you with the knowledge and tools to optimize your health. We'll break down complex concepts into easily digestible information, making it easy to understand and apply. Here's a preview of what you'll discover:

- **Decoding HRV: The Basics and Importance**: We'll start with the fundamentals—what HRV is, why it matters, and how to interpret the numbers. You'll learn how HRV serves as a mirror to your autonomic nervous system and what it reveals about your stress and recovery status.

- **Practical Insights into HRV Monitoring**: Next, we dive into the practicalities of monitoring HRV. You'll get tips on the best tools and practices to track your HRV accurately and learn about the various factors influencing your readings.

- **Habits & Factors that Influence HRV:** Then we'll look at 21 habits and factors that impact your HRV. You'll learn which behaviors have a positive (or negative) impact on your HRV and learn strategies to improve your numbers. This section isn't one you'll necessarily read from start to finish—you'll rapidly learn there is substantial interconnectedness between the aspects discussed. It is intended as a guide you can return to as you begin to take control of your HRV.

- **Creating Your HRV Improvement Plan**: Armed with

your HRV data and the knowledge you've gained, we'll guide you through developing a personalized plan to enhance your HRV. You'll discover lifestyle changes, nutritional adjustments, and exercise strategies to boost your HRV.

Why HRV Matters

So why do you think you should care about HRV? Imagine having a real-time feedback system that tells you how well your body handles stress and recovery. HRV provides this insight, helping you make informed decisions about your training intensity, recovery periods, and sleep quality. Paying attention to HRV can prevent overtraining, reduce the risk of injury, and improve your overall performance and health.

HRV isn't limited to elite athletes. It's a valuable tool for anyone seeking to improve their health, regardless of their fitness level. Whether you're a weekend warrior, a busy professional, or someone striving for better well-being, understanding your HRV can lead to more personalized and effective health strategies.

The Benefits of Reading This Book

By the end of this book, you'll have a comprehensive understanding of HRV and how to use it to your advantage. You'll be equipped with the knowledge to monitor your HRV effectively and make lifestyle changes that enhance your health and performance. Imagine being able to fine-tune your daily habits to optimize your stress levels, recovery, and overall vitality. That's the power of HRV, which this book aims to unlock for you.

A Journey of Discovery

As we embark on this journey together, remember that every small change you make can significantly impact you. This book is designed to be your companion, providing clear, actionable advice every step of the way. We'll debunk myths, clarify complex concepts, and offer practical tips to help you integrate HRV monitoring into your daily routine seamlessly. Rest assured, we'll guide you through every step, making the process as straightforward as possible.

So, let's get started! In the next chapter, we'll dive into the basics of HRV, exploring what it is and why it's such a crucial biomarker. By understanding the fundamentals, you'll be better prepared to make the most of the insights and advice in the subsequent chapters. Welcome to the exciting world of HRV—let's unlock its potential together!

Chapter One

Decoding HRV: The Basics and Importance

Let's get started with the basics—what HRV is, why it's important, and how to interpret the numbers. You'll learn how HRV reflects your autonomic nervous system and what it reveals about your stress and recovery levels.

What is HRV? An Introduction to Heart Rate Variability

Heart Rate Variability (HRV) might sound complex, but it's simply the variation in time between each heartbeat. Think of it as the rhythm and flow of your heart's beats, varying from one beat to the next. Imagine your heart as an orchestra, with each beat representing a note.

The symphony becomes richer and more dynamic when the musicians can skillfully vary their tempo. Similarly, higher HRV generally indicates a more adaptable and resilient cardiovascular system.

HRV balances your autonomic nervous system's sympathetic and parasympathetic branches. The sympathetic branch is like the accelerator, preparing your body for 'fight or flight' responses during stress or physical activity. In contrast, the parasympathetic branch acts as the brake, promoting 'rest and digest' functions that help your body recover and relax. A higher HRV signifies that your body can easily switch between these states, adapting to varying demands and stresses.

Higher HRV often means better cardiovascular fitness and resilience to stress. It indicates that your heart can respond swiftly to changes in your environment, enhancing your overall health and performance. Athletes use HRV to fine-tune their training regimes, ensuring they push their limits without overtraining. But HRV isn't just for athletes—anyone can benefit from understanding and monitoring this vital biomarker. Paying attention to your HRV gives you a deeper insight into your body's internal state, helping you make informed decisions about your health and lifestyle.

Understanding the Autonomic Nervous System's Role in HRV

The autonomic nervous system (ANS) is your body's autopilot, managing essential functions like heart rate, digestion, and respiratory rate without you even thinking about it. It's divided into two main parts: the sympathetic nervous system and the parasympathetic nervous system. Understanding how these two systems interact is critical to grasping the significance of HRV.

The sympathetic nervous system is often called the "fight or flight" system. It prepares your body to handle stressful situations by increasing your heart rate, directing blood flow to muscles, and releasing stress hormones like adrenaline. This response is crucial for survival, allowing you to react quickly to immediate threats or challenges.

On the other hand, the parasympathetic nervous system is known as the "rest and digest" system. It promotes relaxation, recovery, and digestion. When this system is active, your heart rate slows, your blood pressure decreases, and your body can focus on healing and maintenance functions.

HRV provides a window into how well these two systems balance their act. High HRV indicates that your body can efficiently switch between the sympathetic and parasympathetic states, effortlessly adapting to different demands. This flexibility is a sign of a healthy, resilient cardiovascular system.

When you're stressed, the sympathetic nervous system takes over, causing a decrease in HRV. This is because your body is in a heightened state of alertness, ready to respond to perceived threats. Conversely, when relaxed, the parasympathetic nervous system dominates, increasing HRV. This reflects a state of calm and recovery, where your body can perform essential maintenance functions.

By monitoring HRV, you can gain insights into how well your autonomic nervous system functions and responds to stressors. Understanding this balance can help you make informed decisions about managing stress, improving recovery, and optimizing overall health.

HRV as a Health Gauge: What Your Numbers Say

Your HRV numbers can tell you a lot about your overall health. Generally, higher HRV is associated with greater fitness levels, better stress management, and quicker recovery from workouts. Think of HRV as a dynamic health gauge, providing real-time insights into how your body functions and responds to various stressors.

When you consistently see higher HRV readings, it indicates that your body is balanced, effectively managing the demands placed on it. This typically correlates with better cardiovascular fitness, robust autonomic nervous system function, and a greater ability to handle stress. Higher HRV means your body is more adaptable and able to switch efficiently between states of activity and rest, which is crucial for maintaining optimal health.

On the flip side, consistently low HRV can be a warning sign. It might indicate chronic stress, fatigue, or overtraining, signaling that your body struggles to cope with ongoing demands. Low HRV can also be associated with various health issues, such as cardiovascular diseases, metabolic disorders, and psychological stress. Monitoring your HRV can help you detect these potential problems early and take corrective action.

By watching your HRV, you get real-time feedback on how your body copes with stress and recovery. This allows you to adjust your lifestyle and habits to enhance your well-being. For example, if you notice a drop in your HRV, it might be a sign to incorporate more rest days into your workout routine, practice stress-reducing techniques, or improve your sleep hygiene.

HRV serves as a personalized health gauge, guiding you toward better lifestyle choices. By regularly monitoring and interpreting your HRV data, you can proactively manage your health, optimize your performance, and improve your overall quality of life.

The Science of Stress and Recovery Through HRV Lens

Stress is an inevitable part of life, but how you manage it makes all the difference. HRV provides crucial insight into your stress levels and the effectiveness of your recovery processes. Understanding the relationship between stress, recovery, and HRV, you can better manage your daily habits to maintain optimal health and performance.

When stressed, your HRV drops because your body enters a 'fight or flight' mode, dominated by the sympathetic nervous system. This response is essential for handling immediate threats, but prolonged activation can lead to chronic stress, fatigue, and various health problems. During periods of stress, your heart rate tends to become more regular, reducing the variability between beats—a clear indicator of sympathetic dominance.

On the other hand, recovery is marked by an increase in HRV as your body shifts to the 'rest and digest' mode, governed by the parasympathetic nervous system. This state allows your body to repair tissues, replenish energy stores, and perform other essential maintenance functions. A higher HRV during recovery signifies that your body is efficiently managing stress, well-rested, and ready to face new challenges.

Understanding this cycle of stress and recovery is critical to fine-tuning your daily habits. By monitoring your HRV, you can determine whether your body is in a stressed state or recovering effectively. If your HRV remains low over an extended period, it may be a sign that you need to incorporate more rest, relaxation, and stress management techniques into your routine.

Incorporating activities that promote parasympathetic activation—such as mindfulness meditation, deep breathing exercises, yoga, and adequate sleep—can help increase your HRV and enhance your recovery. Balancing periods of intense activity with sufficient downtime ensures that you're not just pushing hard but also giving your body the necessary time to bounce back stronger.

By leveraging HRV to gauge your stress and recovery, you can make informed decisions about your lifestyle and training. This approach helps you maintain a healthy balance, improve your resilience to stress, and optimize your overall well-being.

Debunking HRV Myths: Separating Fact from Fiction

Many misconceptions about HRV exist, so let's set the record straight.

Myth One: "High HRV is always better."

While it is generally true that higher HRV is a sign of good health and adaptability, context matters. An abnormally high HRV can sometimes indicate overtraining or illness. For example, suppose your HRV spikes unusually high without corresponding changes in your routine. In that case, it might be a sign that your body is under more stress than you realize, potentially from an underlying condition. Always consider your HRV readings within the broader context of your overall health and any other symptoms you may be experiencing.

Myth Two: "Only athletes need to monitor HRV."

Not so! HRV is valuable for anyone looking to optimize their health and stress management. While athletes use HRV to fine-tune their training and recovery, others can benefit just as much. HRV provides insights into how well your body handles stress, recovers from daily activities, and maintains balance. Whether managing a high-stress job, aiming to improve your fitness, or wanting to enhance your overall well-being, monitoring HRV can provide actionable insights that help you make better lifestyle choices.

Myth Three: "HRV is too complex to understand."

With the right tools and a bit of knowledge, interpreting HRV is straightforward and immensely beneficial for everyone. Modern HRV monitoring devices and apps make tracking and understanding your HRV easy. These tools often provide user-friendly interfaces and explanations, helping you interpret your data without needing an advanced degree. By learning the basics and regularly monitoring your HRV, you can gain valuable insights into your health and make informed decisions to improve your well-being.

By debunking these common myths, we hope to make HRV more accessible and encourage you to incorporate it into your health monitoring routine. Understanding and leveraging HRV can empower you to take proactive steps towards a healthier, more balanced life.

By the end of this chapter, you should have a solid understanding of what HRV is, why it's essential, and how you can start using this vital biomarker to enhance your health and well-being. Next, we'll dive into monitoring your HRV, examining tools and practices to track your HRV accurately and learn about the various factors influencing your readings.

Chapter Two
Practical Insights into HRV Monitoring

In this chapter, we'll explain what HRV is, why it's important, and how to interpret the numbers. You'll discover how HRV reflects the state of your autonomic nervous system and what it indicates about your stress and recovery levels.

Choosing the Right HRV Monitoring Device

When monitoring HRV, the device you choose is not just a tool; it's a crucial part of your health strategy. With many options available, finding the perfect fit for your needs can be overwhelming. But fear not; here's a guide to help you select a reliable and accurate measurement device, giving you the confidence that you're making the right choice.

Chest Strap Monitors

Chest strap monitors, such as the Polar H10, are renowned for their precision and are considered the gold standard for HRV measurement. These devices provide consistent, high-quality data by directly measuring electrical signals from the heart. They are especially favored by serious athletes and those who require the utmost accuracy in their HRV readings.

Advanced Wearables

Advanced wearables like the Whoop Strap, some fitness watches and the Oura Ring offer continuous HRV monitoring with minimal fuss for everyday convenience. These devices are designed to be worn comfortably throughout the day and night, providing seamless tracking of your HRV without being intrusive. They sync with dedicated apps that analyze your data, offering insights into your recovery status, stress levels, and overall health trends.

Compatibility with HRV-Specific Apps

Make sure the device you choose is compatible with HRV-specific apps. Apps like Elite HRV, HRV4Training, or Whoop's app provide in-depth analysis and tracking features to help you understand your HRV data. These apps often offer additional functionalities such as trend analysis, personalized insights, and recommendations based on your HRV metrics.

When selecting a device, consider factors such as comfort, battery life, data accuracy, and the availability of comprehensive analysis tools. Whether you opt for a chest strap or a wearable, ensure it aligns with your lifestyle and health goals. A well-chosen HRV monitoring device can be a game-changer, providing the data you need to optimize your training, recovery, and overall well-being.

Interpreting Your HRV Scores: A Beginner's Guide

Interpreting HRV scores might seem daunting initially, but rest assured, you'll quickly get the hang of it with some guidance. HRV is typically measured in milliseconds, and a higher number generally indicates better autonomic nervous system balance and overall health. Let's break down the basics to help you understand and use your HRV data effectively, making the process less intimidating.

Understanding the Numbers

HRV is measured by the variation in time intervals between heartbeats, often in milliseconds. Most apps and devices will present your HRV data in a user-friendly format, providing a daily score and trends over time. A higher HRV score typically suggests that your body is well-balanced and can adapt to stress efficiently. In comparison, a lower HRV score may indicate stress, fatigue, or inadequate recovery.

Establishing a Baseline

When you start tracking your HRV, the first step is to establish a baseline. This is your average HRV over some time, usually a few weeks. Your baseline serves as a reference point to compare daily readings. Most HRV monitoring apps will help you calculate this baseline and use it to interpret your scores. Establishing a baseline is crucial as it provides a context for your daily HRV readings and enables you to understand if your HRV is improving or declining over time.

Focusing on Trends

While daily HRV readings are essential, observing trends over time is the actual value. Pay attention to how your HRV changes day-to-day and week-to-week. A single low reading might not be a cause for concern, but a gradual decline in HRV over several days can signal accumulating stress or inadequate recovery. Conversely, a consistent upward trend indicates improved autonomic nervous system balance and overall health.

Making Adjustments Based on HRV Trends

If you notice a decline in your HRV, it may be time to adjust your lifestyle habits. This could mean incorporating more rest days into your workout routine, practicing stress management techniques, or improving your sleep hygiene. For example, if you see a drop in HRV following intense exercise sessions, consider increasing your recovery time. Similarly, if stress from work is affecting your HRV, integrating mindfulness practices or relaxation techniques can help.

Using HRV Apps and Tools

Most HRV apps and devices have features to help you interpret your data. They often provide insights and recommendations based on your HRV trends. Utilize these tools to understand better how different activities, stressors, and recovery practices impact your HRV. Many apps offer community support and educational resources to enhance your HRV knowledge. HRV apps and tools play a significant role in HRV monitoring. They provide detailed analysis, personalized insights, and recommendations based on your HRV data, enhancing your HRV tracking experience.

Regularly monitoring and interpreting your HRV scores gives you a powerful tool to make informed decisions about your health and lifestyle. This understanding empowers you to proactively manage stress, optimize recovery, and maintain overall well-being, putting you in the driver's seat of your health journey.

Common Mistakes in HRV Measurement and How to Avoid Them

To ensure accurate HRV readings, it's essential to avoid common pitfalls. Here are some tips to help you get the most reliable data:

1. Consistency is Key

Measure your HRV at the same time each day, ideally in the morning before getting out of bed. This reduces the impact of daily fluctuations caused by activity, meals, or stress. Morning measurements provide a consistent baseline, reflecting your body's natural state before external factors come into play.

2. Stay Still During Measurements

Movement can cause inaccuracies in your HRV readings. Ensure you are completely still during the measurement process. This helps your device capture the precise intervals between heartbeats without interference from motion, which can lead to erroneous data.

3. Proper Device Positioning

Ensure your device is positioned correctly and has a good connection. Correct placement is crucial, whether using a chest strap or a wearable device. Follow the manufacturer's instructions to place the device accurately and securely. Ensure chest straps are snug against your skin and properly aligned. For wearables, ensure they are tight enough to maintain contact without being uncomfortable.

4. Avoid Immediate Post-Exercise, Caffeine, or Stressful Events

Avoid taking readings immediately after intense exercise, caffeine intake, or stressful events, as these can temporarily skew your HRV. Intense physical activity can elevate your heart rate and reduce HRV temporarily. Similarly, caffeine and stress can cause short-term fluctuations. To get an accurate picture of your baseline HRV, measure it in a calm, relaxed state.

5. Maintain a Routine

Establish a routine with a set time and environment for your HRV measurements. Consistency in your measurement routine helps in minimizing variables that can affect HRV. This practice allows for more accurate tracking of trends and changes over time.

6. Calibrate Your Device Regularly

Ensure your device is functioning correctly by calibrating it regularly, if applicable. Some devices may require periodic calibration to maintain accuracy. Check the manufacturer's recommendations for keeping your device.

By following these guidelines, you'll obtain more reliable HRV data. Accurate HRV readings are essential for making informed decisions about your health and lifestyle, helping you optimize your well-being and performance.

The Best Times to Measure HRV for Optimal Insights

Timing is everything when it comes to HRV measurement. The best time to measure HRV is first thing in the morning, right after waking up. This is when your body is most rested, providing a clear picture of your baseline autonomic function. Morning measurements are less likely to be influenced by daily activities or stressors, offering a consistent snapshot of your HRV.

Morning HRV readings are beneficial because they reflect your body's recovery from the previous day's activities and stressors. This time of day provides a reliable baseline that helps you understand how well your autonomic nervous system functions without interference from daily fluctuations.

Some devices also allow for nighttime HRV monitoring, which can provide additional insights into your sleep quality and recovery. Nighttime measurements track your HRV throughout different sleep stages, giving you a comprehensive view of how well your body is resting and recovering during sleep. This can be especially useful for identifying patterns related to sleep disorders or disturbances affecting your overall health.

Consistent measurement times will help you track trends more accurately, making it easier to identify patterns and make informed adjustments to your routine. Consistency is vital whether you measure HRV in the morning or utilize nighttime monitoring. Stick to the same time frame daily to ensure your data remains reliable and comparable.

Maintaining a consistent measurement schedule, you can better understand the factors that influence your HRV and make targeted changes to improve your overall well-being. Regular monitoring and timely adjustments based on your HRV trends will help you optimize your health and performance, ensuring your body remains resilient and adaptable to various stressors.

Long-term HRV Tracking: Trends You Should Watch

Monitoring HRV over the long term can reveal significant trends that inform your health strategies. Keep an eye on sustained increases or decreases in your baseline HRV. An upward trend generally indicates improved fitness, better stress management, and enhanced recovery, while a downward trend might suggest overtraining, chronic stress, or poor sleep quality. Use your HRV data to identify how habits and lifestyle changes impact your health. For example, you might notice that incorporating regular meditation sessions boosts your HRV or that certain foods negatively affect your readings. Observing these trends lets you fine-tune your daily routines to optimize your health and performance.

With these practical insights into HRV monitoring, you can effectively measure and interpret your HRV. Avoid common mistakes, choose the correct times for measurement, and focus on long-term trends to better understand your health. Let's dive deeper into this fascinating topic and discover how small changes in your daily habits can significantly improve your HRV and overall health.

Chapter Three

Habits & Factors that Influence HRV

This section empowers you with knowledge about 21 essential habits and factors that directly influence your HRV, such as stress, diet, physical activity, sleep quality, hydration, and age. By understanding these, you can make informed choices about your lifestyle. You'll gain insights into which behaviors, like deep breathing, yoga, and mindfulness meditation, can either boost or hinder your HRV. Most importantly, you'll discover practical strategies to enhance your HRV scores, giving you a sense of control and hope for a healthier life.

Each factor is presented individually with optimization tips, making this section a valuable reference.

If you read this section in one go, you'll quickly notice the significant overlap and interrelation between many factors. This interconnectedness is a testament to the complexity and importance of our habits and factors in influencing HRV. Let's begin our exploration!

Stress

Picture this: you're in a high-pressure situation. Your heart starts pounding, your breaths become shallow, and you feel a sudden surge of energy. This is your body's 'fight or flight' response, a natural stress-related reaction. While this response is essential for dealing with immediate threats, it can be harmful if it persists. Chronic stress can keep your body in a constant state of alert, leading to consistently low HRV, which is a measure of the variation in time between each heartbeat, indicating that your body struggles to cope effectively.

Now that we understand the impact of stress on HRV let's explore some practical strategies to manage it. These strategies are like a lifeline in your stress management toolkit, ready to be used whenever needed. Here are a few techniques you can start incorporating into your daily routine, bringing a sense of relief and hope for better HRV:

Deep Breathing Exercises

Deep breathing can help activate the parasympathetic nervous system, a part of your autonomic nervous system that helps your body rest and digest, promoting relaxation and increasing HRV. Techniques such as diaphragmatic breathing or box breathing can be particularly effective. Set aside a few minutes each day to focus on slow, deep breaths, inhaling through your nose, holding for a few seconds, and exhaling slowly through your mouth.

Yoga

Yoga is a powerful tool that combines physical postures, breathing exercises, and meditation. It's an excellent practice for reducing stress and improving HRV. Regular yoga sessions can help balance your autonomic nervous system, enhance relaxation, and increase your HRV. Incorporate yoga into your weekly routine and start reaping its benefits, feeling motivated and encouraged on your HRV improvement journey.

Mindfulness Meditation

Mindfulness meditation involves focusing on the present moment and accepting it without judgment. This practice has been shown to reduce stress, lower cortisol levels, and increase HRV. Start with short sessions, gradually increasing the duration as you become more comfortable with the practice. Use guided meditations or mindfulness apps to help you get started.

Prioritize Relaxation

Make relaxation a priority in your daily life. Engage in calming and enjoyable activities, whether reading, listening to music, spending time in nature, or practicing a hobby. Regularly taking time to unwind can help reduce stress levels and improve your HRV.

Regular Physical Activity

While intense exercise can temporarily lower HRV, regular moderate physical activity can enhance your overall stress resilience and improve HRV over time. Aim for a balanced exercise routine that includes both aerobic and anaerobic activities, and ensure you allow adequate recovery time.

Incorporating these stress management techniques into your daily routine can significantly improve your HRV and overall well-being. By understanding the impact of stress on your HRV and taking proactive steps to manage it, you're not just maintaining a healthier, more balanced life, but also empowering yourself to take control of your health. This knowledge and action give you hope for a better future, where you can navigate stress with confidence and resilience.

Diet

What you eat can have a profound impact on your HRV. A diet rich in whole foods, including fruits, vegetables, lean proteins, and healthy fats, supports better HRV. Here's how to optimize your diet for improved heart rate variability:

Whole Foods

Focus on consuming a variety of whole foods. These include fresh fruits and vegetables, whole grains, lean proteins, nuts, seeds, and healthy fats. Whole foods provide essential nutrients that support overall health and autonomic nervous system function, contributing to higher HRV.

Avoid Processed Foods

Avoid excessive consumption of processed foods, sugars, and unhealthy fats. These can negatively affect your HRV by promoting inflammation, a process in which your body's white blood cells protect you from infection, but can also damage your heart and blood vessels, increasing oxidative stress, a condition in which your body doesn't have enough antioxidants to neutralize the free radicals, and disrupting metabolic processes. Foods high in refined sugars and trans fats can lead to spikes in blood sugar and increase stress on your cardiovascular system, resulting in lower HRV.

Omega-3 Fatty Acids

Incorporate foods rich in omega-3 fatty acids, such as fish (salmon, mackerel, sardines), flaxseed, chia seeds, and walnuts. Omega-3s are known for their anti-inflammatory properties and ability to improve heart health. Regular intake of these fatty acids has been shown to enhance HRV by supporting cardiovascular function and reducing systemic inflammation.

Balanced Diet

Ensure your diet includes balanced macronutrients—carbohydrates, proteins, and fats. Each plays a role in maintaining energy levels, supporting bodily functions, and promoting recovery. Aim for complex carbohydrates (like whole grains and legumes), lean proteins (like chicken, fish, and plant-based options), and healthy fats (like avocados, nuts, and olive oil).

Regular Eating Schedule

Maintain a regular eating schedule to help regulate your body's metabolic processes and support steady energy levels. Eating at consistent times can help stabilize your blood sugar levels, reduce stress on your digestive system, and improve your HRV. Try to avoid skipping meals or eating at irregular intervals.

Avoid Heavy Meals Before Bedtime

Avoid heavy meals before bedtime, as they can disrupt your sleep and negatively impact your HRV. Your body needs time to digest food, and eating large meals late at night can lead to discomfort, impaired sleep quality, and reduced HRV. Aim to have your last meal at least 2-3 hours before bed to ensure proper digestion and restful sleep.

These dietary guidelines can support your autonomic nervous system, reduce stress, and improve your HRV. Making mindful food choices and maintaining a balanced, nutrient-rich diet will improve overall health and well-being.

Physical Activity

Regular physical activity is not just beneficial; it's crucial for maintaining and improving HRV. Exercise is a powerful tool that helps to balance the autonomic nervous system, enhancing HRV over time. By engaging in aerobic and anaerobic exercises, you're not just improving your heart rate variability significantly, but also committing to a healthier lifestyle. This understanding should inspire and motivate you to prioritize physical activity in your life.

Aerobic Exercises

Aerobic exercises like running, swimming, cycling, and brisk walking boost HRV. These activities improve cardiovascular fitness by enhancing the efficiency of your heart and lungs, promoting better oxygen delivery to your muscles and organs. As health guidelines recommend, aim for at least 150 minutes of moderate aerobic activity or 75 minutes of vigorous aerobic activity per week.

Anaerobic Exercises

Anaerobic exercises, including weightlifting, high-intensity interval training (HIIT), and resistance training, are essential for improving HRV. These exercises help build muscle strength, improve metabolic health, and enhance your body's ability to handle short bursts of intense effort. Incorporate anaerobic exercises into your routine 2-3 times weekly for optimal benefits.

Avoiding Overtraining

While regular physical activity is essential, it's important to avoid overtraining, which can lead to excessive physical stress and lower HRV. Overtraining occurs when you push your body too hard without allowing adequate recovery time, resulting in fatigue, decreased performance, and increased risk of injury. Monitor your HRV to ensure you're not overtraining—if you notice a consistent decline in HRV, it may be time to incorporate more rest and recovery days.

Balancing Intensity and Recovery

To keep your HRV at optimal levels, incorporate high-intensity workouts, moderate exercises, and recovery days. High-intensity workouts can boost your cardiovascular and muscular strength, but they should be balanced with moderate exercises that promote endurance and overall fitness. Recovery days, including light activities like walking or yoga, are crucial for allowing your body to rest, repair, and rejuvenate.

Listening to Your Body

Pay attention to your body's signals and adjust your exercise routine accordingly. If you're feeling fatigued or notice a drop in your HRV, it might be a sign to reduce the intensity or duration of your workouts and focus on recovery. Consistently high HRV readings indicate that your body responds well to your exercise regimen, while low readings can alert you to potential overtraining or the need for more rest.

By incorporating a balanced exercise routine that includes aerobic and anaerobic activities, avoiding overtraining, and allowing for adequate recovery, you can significantly improve your HRV and overall health. Regular physical activity enhances your fitness and promotes a healthier, more resilient autonomic nervous system.

Sleep Quality

Quality sleep is essential for a healthy HRV. During sleep, your body undergoes repair and recovery processes crucial for maintaining high HRV. Here's how to optimize your sleep to enhance HRV and overall well-being:

Aim for 7-9 Hours of Sleep

Most adults need 7-9 hours of sleep per night to support optimal health. This range allows your body enough time to cycle through the various stages of sleep, including deep sleep and REM sleep, which are vital for physical and mental recovery.

Maintain a Consistent Sleep Schedule

Going to bed and waking up at the same time daily helps regulate your body's internal clock, also known as the circadian rhythm. A consistent sleep schedule improves the quality of your sleep and helps stabilize your HRV. Try to stick to this routine even on weekends to reinforce your body's natural sleep-wake cycle.

Create a Sleep-Friendly Environment

Your sleep environment plays a significant role in the quality of your sleep. Ensure your bedroom is conducive to rest by keeping it cool, dark, and quiet. A room temperature between 60-67°F (15-19°C) is ideal for most people. Use blackout curtains or a sleep mask to block out light, and consider using earplugs or a white noise machine to minimize disturbances from noise.

Avoid Screens Before Bedtime

Exposure to the blue light emitted by screens (phones, tablets, computers, and TVs) can interfere with your body's production of melatonin, the hormone that regulates sleep. Aim to turn off electronic devices at least an hour before bed. Instead, engage in relaxing activities such as reading a book, listening to calming music, or practicing meditation.

Limit Caffeine and Alcohol Intake

Caffeine is a stimulant that can disrupt your sleep if consumed too late in the day. Try to avoid caffeine at least 6 hours before bedtime. Similarly, while alcohol might help you fall asleep faster, it can disrupt your sleep cycle and negatively impact your HRV. Limit alcohol consumption, especially close to bedtime.

Practice Good Sleep Hygiene

Good sleep hygiene involves adopting habits that promote consistent, uninterrupted sleep. This includes keeping your sleep environment clean and comfortable, using your bed only for sleep and sex (not for working or watching TV), and establishing a relaxing pre-sleep routine to signal your body that it's time to wind down.

Manage Stress and Anxiety

Stress and anxiety can significantly interfere with your ability to fall and stay asleep. Incorporate stress management techniques such as deep breathing exercises, mindfulness meditation, and progressive muscle relaxation into your bedtime routine to help calm your mind and prepare your body for sleep.

By prioritizing quality sleep and practicing good sleep hygiene, you can significantly enhance your HRV and overall health. A well-rested body is better equipped to handle stress, recover from physical exertion, and maintain optimal autonomic nervous system function.

Hydration

Staying well-hydrated is vital for optimal HRV. Dehydration can negatively impact cardiovascular function and lower HRV. Proper hydration supports the efficient regulation of your autonomic nervous system, which is crucial for maintaining a healthy HRV.

The Importance of Hydration

Hydration plays a critical role in maintaining cardiovascular health. Water is essential for your heart, blood vessels, and muscles to function correctly. It helps in the transport of nutrients and oxygen to cells, the removal of waste products, and the regulation of body temperature. When you're dehydrated, your body has to work harder to perform these functions, which can lead to increased stress and lower HRV.

Daily Water Intake

Make sure to drink enough water throughout the day to stay well-hydrated. The water you need can vary based on age, weight, activity level, and climate. A general guideline is to aim for at least eight 8-ounce glasses of water daily, but you may need more if you're physically active or live in a hot climate.

Monitoring Hydration Levels

One of the simplest ways to monitor your hydration levels is by checking the color of your urine. Pale yellow urine typically indicates proper hydration, while dark yellow or amber urine suggests that you may need to drink more water. Make it a habit to check your urine color throughout the day and adjust your water intake accordingly.

Hydration During Physical Activity

If you're physically active, it's imperative to stay hydrated. Exercise increases your body's need for water as you lose fluids through sweat. Drink water before, during, and after exercise to maintain hydration levels. For lengthier or more intense workouts, consider sports drinks containing electrolytes to replenish the minerals lost through sweat.

Other Hydration Tips

- **Start Your Day with Water:** Start each day by drinking water to kickstart your hydration.

- **Carry a Water Bottle:** Keep a reusable water bottle with you throughout the day as a reminder to drink regularly.

- **Eat Water-Rich Foods:** Incorporate water-rich foods like fruits and vegetables (e.g., cucumbers, oranges, and watermelon) into your diet to boost your hydration.

- **Limit Dehydrating Beverages:** Reduce your intake of caffeinated and alcoholic beverages, which can contribute to dehydration.

Maintaining adequate hydration supports your body's ability to regulate autonomic function effectively. Proper hydration not only helps in sustaining high HRV but also contributes to overall health and well-being.

Age

Age naturally affects HRV, with younger individuals typically having higher HRV than older adults. This variation is due to several factors related to aging, including cardiovascular and autonomic nervous system changes.

Natural Decline in HRV with Age

As we age, the responsiveness of the autonomic nervous system decreases, leading to lower HRV. This decline is partly due to the reduced elasticity of the heart and blood vessels and changes in the nervous system's regulation. Younger individuals generally have a more adaptable and resilient autonomic nervous system, reflected in higher HRV scores.

Mitigating Age-Related Declines in HRV

While it's natural for HRV to decrease with age, there are several ways to mitigate this decline through lifestyle choices:

- **Regular Exercise:** Regular physical activity is one of the most effective ways to maintain higher HRV levels as you age.

Aerobic exercises (like walking, running, and swimming) and anaerobic exercises (like weightlifting and high-intensity interval training) can improve cardiovascular health and enhance autonomic function. Exercise helps keep the heart and blood vessels healthy, promoting better HRV.

- **Stress Management:** Effective stress management is crucial for maintaining high HRV levels. Chronic stress can accelerate the decline in HRV, making it essential to incorporate stress-reducing activities into your routine. Meditation, yoga, deep breathing exercises, and mindfulness can help manage stress and support autonomic balance.

- **Healthy Lifestyle Choices:** Adopting a healthy lifestyle can significantly impact HRV. This includes maintaining a balanced diet rich in whole foods, staying well-hydrated, getting adequate sleep, and avoiding harmful habits like smoking and excessive alcohol consumption. A healthy lifestyle supports overall cardiovascular health and helps maintain higher HRV levels.

- **Staying Active and Engaged:** Remaining physically and socially active can also improve HRV. Regular physical activity keeps your body fit, while social engagement and mental stimulation support mental and emotional health. Both aspects are essential for maintaining a resilient autonomic nervous system.

Monitoring HRV as You Age

Regularly monitoring your HRV can provide valuable insights into how your body responds to aging and your lifestyle choices. Use this information to adjust as needed, ensuring you continue supporting your autonomic health. If you notice significant changes in your HRV, it may be worth consulting a healthcare professional for personalized advice.

By staying active, managing stress, and making healthy lifestyle choices, you can mitigate age-related declines in HRV and maintain better overall health. These efforts will help preserve your autonomic function and enhance your quality of life as you age.

Genetics

Genetics plays a role in determining baseline HRV levels. Some people naturally have higher or lower HRV due to their genetic makeup. While you can't change your genetics, understanding your baseline can help you make informed decisions about lifestyle changes that can optimize your HRV.

The Role of Genetics in HRV

Research indicates that genetic factors contribute significantly to HRV. These genetic influences affect how your autonomic nervous system responds to stress and recovery. Consequently, some individuals may have inherently higher or lower HRV readings, which are reflective of their genetic predisposition.

Understanding Your Baseline

To make the most of HRV monitoring, it's essential to understand your baseline HRV. This baseline represents your average HRV over a period of time, accounting for your unique genetic makeup. By establishing your baseline, you can better interpret daily fluctuations and trends in your HRV, helping you to distinguish between normal variations and significant changes that might require attention.

Making Informed Lifestyle Changes

Even though you can't change your genetics, you can optimize your HRV by making informed lifestyle changes. Regular monitoring of your HRV can guide you in identifying which habits and interventions are most effective for improving your autonomic function. For example:

- **Exercise:** Tailor your exercise routine to include both aerobic and anaerobic activities, and ensure you allow for adequate recovery.

- **Diet:** Focus on a balanced diet rich in whole foods, and avoid processed foods that can negatively impact your HRV.

- **Stress Management:** Incorporate stress-reducing activities such as meditation, yoga, and deep breathing exercises into your daily routine.

- **Sleep:** Prioritize quality sleep by maintaining a consistent sleep schedule and practicing good sleep hygiene.

- **Hydration:** Ensure you stay well-hydrated throughout the day to support cardiovascular function.

Regular Monitoring and Adjustment

Regularly monitoring your HRV lets you track how your body responds to various lifestyle changes. Use this data to adjust your habits and optimize your routine for better HRV. By staying consistent with your monitoring and being proactive in making adjustments, you can significantly improve your HRV, regardless of your genetic predisposition.

Personalizing Your Approach

Understanding that genetics play a role in HRV can also help you personalize your approach to health and wellness. Accept that factors beyond your control influence your baseline HRV and focus on the aspects you can influence. This personalized approach ensures you set realistic goals and maintain a positive outlook toward better health.

By acknowledging the role of genetics and taking a proactive approach to monitoring and optimizing your HRV, you can make meaningful improvements in your autonomic health and overall well-being. Embrace your unique baseline as a foundation for informed decision-making and lifestyle adjustments.

Medical Conditions

Certain medical conditions, such as cardiovascular diseases, diabetes, and chronic illnesses, can significantly affect HRV. Understanding and managing these conditions is crucial for optimizing HRV and improving overall health. Here's how different medical conditions impact HRV and what you can do to manage them effectively:

Cardiovascular Diseases

Conditions like hypertension, coronary artery disease, and heart failure can lower HRV. These conditions strain the heart and the autonomic nervous system, reducing heart rate variability. To manage cardiovascular diseases and improve HRV, follow these steps:

- **Medication:** Take prescribed medications as directed by your healthcare provider to control blood pressure, cholesterol levels, and heart function.

- **Lifestyle Changes:** Adopt a heart-healthy diet, engage in regular physical activity, avoid smoking, and limit alcohol consumption.

- **Regular Check-Ups:** Schedule regular medical check-ups

to monitor your heart health and adjust your treatment plan as needed.

Diabetes

Diabetes, particularly when poorly managed, can lead to autonomic neuropathy, a condition that damages the nerves controlling heart rate, resulting in lower HRV. To manage diabetes and support HRV:

- **Blood Sugar Control:** Use medication, diet, and exercise to keep your blood sugar levels within the target range.

- **Healthy Diet:** Follow a balanced diet rich in whole foods and low in refined sugars and unhealthy fats.

- **Physical Activity:** Exercise regularly to improve insulin sensitivity and cardiovascular health.

- **Regular Monitoring:** Monitor your blood sugar levels regularly and consult your healthcare provider to adjust your treatment plan.

Chronic Illnesses

Chronic illnesses such as chronic obstructive pulmonary disease (COPD), chronic kidney disease, and autoimmune disorders can also impact HRV. Managing these conditions involves:

- **Medication Adherence:** Take medications as prescribed to control symptoms and prevent complications.

- **Lifestyle Adjustments:** Make necessary changes to manage your condition, such as dietary modifications, exercise, and stress management.

- **Medical Supervision:** Regularly visit your healthcare provider to monitor your condition and adjust your treatment plan.

Stress and Mental Health Disorders

Conditions like anxiety and depression can significantly affect HRV by increasing sympathetic nervous system activity and reducing parasympathetic activity. To manage these conditions and improve HRV:

- **Therapy and Counseling:** Seek professional help through therapy or counseling to address underlying issues and develop coping strategies.

- **Medication:** Take prescribed medications as directed to manage symptoms effectively.

- **Stress Management:** Incorporate stress-reducing activities such as mindfulness, meditation, and physical activity into your daily routine.

Collaboration with Healthcare Providers

Working closely with your healthcare provider is essential for managing medical conditions and optimizing HRV. Regular monitoring of your HRV can provide valuable insights into how well your condition is being managed. Your healthcare provider can help you interpret HRV data and make informed decisions about your treatment plan.

Regular Monitoring and Adjustments

Regularly monitor your HRV to track changes and trends. If you notice significant fluctuations, consult your healthcare provider to determine if your treatment plan needs adjustments. Effective management of medical conditions can help stabilize and improve your HRV, contributing to better overall health.

By effectively managing medical conditions through medication, lifestyle changes, and regular check-ups, you can optimize your HRV and enhance your overall well-being. Monitoring HRV provides valuable feedback on how well your treatment plan is working and helps you make informed decisions about your health.

Inflammation

Elevated levels of systemic inflammation are associated with lower HRV. Inflammation is a natural response of the immune system to injury or infection, but chronic inflammation can negatively impact cardiovascular health and autonomic nervous system function, leading to reduced HRV.

Understanding Inflammation and HRV

Inflammation triggers the release of various inflammatory cytokines and other immune mediators. While these responses are essential for fighting infections and healing injuries, chronic inflammation can persist due to poor diet, stress, lack of exercise, and underlying health conditions. This persistent inflammatory state can adversely affect the autonomic nervous system, decreasing HRV.

Causes of Chronic Inflammation

Several lifestyle and environmental factors contribute to chronic inflammation:

- **Diet:** Consuming a diet high in processed foods, sugars, and unhealthy fats can promote inflammation.

- **Stress:** Chronic psychological stress can elevate inflammatory markers in the body.

- **Sedentary Lifestyle:** Lack of physical activity is associated with increased inflammation.

- **Poor Sleep:** Inadequate or poor-quality sleep can elevate inflammatory cytokines.

- **Environmental Toxins:** Exposure to pollutants and toxins can trigger inflammatory responses.

Reducing Inflammation to Improve HRV

To lower inflammation and improve HRV, consider implementing the following strategies:

- **Healthy Diet:** Adopt an anti-inflammatory diet rich in whole foods such as fruits, vegetables, lean proteins, whole grains, and healthy fats. Foods rich in omega-3 fatty acids, like fish, flaxseeds, and walnuts, have anti-inflammatory properties. Additionally, spices like turmeric and ginger are known for their anti-inflammatory effects.

- **Regular Exercise:** Engage in regular physical activity, which has been shown to reduce systemic inflammation. Both aerobic and resistance exercises can help. Aim for at least 150 minutes of moderate-intensity exercise per week.

- **Stress Management:** Practice stress-reducing techniques such as mindfulness meditation, deep breathing exercises, yoga, and progressive muscle relaxation. Managing stress effectively can help lower inflammatory markers and improve HRV.

- **Adequate Sleep:** Ensure you get 7-9 hours of quality sleep per night. Establish a regular sleep schedule and create a sleep-friendly environment to enhance sleep quality. Good sleep hygiene can reduce inflammation and support autonomic balance.

- **Avoid Toxins:** Minimize exposure to environmental toxins by avoiding smoking, limiting alcohol intake, and reducing exposure to pollutants. Use natural cleaning products and ensure good ventilation in your living spaces.

Monitoring Inflammation and HRV

Regularly monitor your HRV to track how lifestyle changes affect your inflammation levels. Improvements in HRV can indicate successful reductions in systemic inflammation. Consult your healthcare provider for tests that measure inflammatory markers, such as C-reactive protein (CRP), to get a clearer picture of your inflammation levels.

Adopting an anti-inflammatory lifestyle and making informed diet, exercise, stress management, and sleep choices can reduce systemic inflammation and improve your HRV. Lowering inflammation enhances HRV and contributes to better overall health and well-being.

Medications

Certain medications, including beta-blockers, ACE inhibitors, antiarrhythmics, and some psychotropic drugs, can affect HRV. Understanding how these medications influence HRV can help you manage your health more effectively, especially if you monitor HRV as part of your wellness routine.

Beta-Blockers

Beta-blockers are commonly prescribed for conditions like hypertension, heart arrhythmias, and anxiety. These medications work by blocking the effects of adrenaline on your heart, which helps to lower heart rate and blood pressure. Beta-blockers can increase HRV by reducing sympathetic nervous system activity and promoting parasympathetic dominance. However, the impact on HRV can vary depending on the specific beta-blocker and the individual's health condition.

ACE Inhibitors

ACE inhibitors treat high blood pressure and heart failure by relaxing blood vessels and reducing the workload on the heart. These medications can positively affect HRV by improving autonomic balance and reducing the strain on the cardiovascular system. By lowering blood pressure and decreasing sympathetic nervous system activity, ACE inhibitors can contribute to higher HRV.

Antiarrhythmics

Antiarrhythmic medications treat irregular heart rhythms by stabilizing the heart's electrical activity. The impact of these medications on HRV can vary depending on the specific drug and the underlying condition being treated. Some antiarrhythmics may improve HRV by reducing abnormal heart rhythms and promoting a more stable autonomic function.

Psychotropic Drugs

Psychotropic drugs, including antidepressants, antipsychotics, and anxiolytics, can also affect HRV. These medications influence neurotransmitter levels in the brain, impacting autonomic nervous system function. For example:

- **Antidepressants:** Selective serotonin reuptake inhibitors (SSRIs) and other antidepressants can have varying effects on HRV. Some studies suggest that certain antidepressants may improve HRV by alleviating symptoms of depression and anxiety, which are associated with lower HRV.

- **Antipsychotics:** Antipsychotic medications can have a significant impact on HRV, often leading to a reduction in HRV due to their effects on autonomic regulation. The degree of impact can depend on the specific drug and dosage.

- **Anxiolytics:** Medications used to treat anxiety, such as benzodiazepines, can affect HRV by altering autonomic balance. While they may reduce acute anxiety and its impact on HRV, long-term use can lead to dependence and other side effects that may negatively affect HRV.

Monitoring and Adjusting Medications

If you take any of these medications, monitoring your HRV regularly and discussing significant changes with your healthcare provider is essential. They can help you understand how your medications affect your HRV and adjust your treatment plan if necessary. Only adjust or discontinue medicines after consulting your healthcare provider, as doing so can have serious health consequences.

Integrating Lifestyle Changes

In addition to medication management, integrating lifestyle changes such as regular exercise, stress management, a healthy diet, and good sleep hygiene can help support optimal HRV. Working closely with your healthcare provider, you can develop a comprehensive approach to managing your health, including medication and lifestyle interventions.

By understanding the impact of medications on HRV and working with your healthcare provider to monitor and adjust your treatment plan, you can optimize your HRV and overall health.

Body Weight

Maintaining a healthy body weight is vital for optimal HRV. Obesity can negatively impact HRV, as excess body weight puts additional strain on the cardiovascular system. Here's how body weight affects HRV and what you can do to achieve and maintain a healthy weight to improve your HRV.

Impact of Obesity on HRV

Obesity is associated with lower HRV, reduced autonomic nervous system flexibility and higher cardiovascular stress. Excess body weight can lead to a variety of health issues, including hypertension, diabetes, and sleep apnea, all of which can further reduce HRV. The additional fat tissue increases the workload on the heart, making it harder for the cardiovascular system to function efficiently.

Benefits of a Healthy Weight

Achieving and maintaining a healthy weight can improve HRV by reducing the strain on your cardiovascular system and enhancing overall autonomic function. A healthy weight supports better blood pressure regulation, improved insulin sensitivity, and reduced inflammation, all contributing to higher HRV.

Strategies for Achieving and Maintaining a Healthy Weight

- **Balanced Diet:** Adopt a balanced diet rich in whole foods, including fruits, vegetables, lean proteins, whole grains, and healthy fats. Avoid excessive consumption of processed foods, sugars, and unhealthy fats. Focus on portion control and mindful eating to support weight management.

- **Regular Exercise:** Regular exercise to help manage your weight and improve HRV. Incorporate aerobic exercises, like walking, running, or swimming, and strength training exercises, like weightlifting or bodyweight workouts. Aim for at least 150 minutes of moderate-intensity aerobic activity per week and muscle-strengthening activities two or more days per week.

- **Monitor Your Weight:** Regularly monitor your weight to track your progress and make necessary adjustments to your diet and exercise routine. Use a reliable scale and keep a record of your weight over time. Monitoring your weight can help you stay accountable and motivated.

- **Gradual, Sustainable Changes:** Focus on making gradual, sustainable changes to your lifestyle rather than quick fixes or extreme diets. Sustainable changes will likely lead to long-term weight management and improved HRV. Set realistic goals and celebrate small milestones along the way.

- **Healthy Habits:** Incorporate healthy habits into your daily routine, such as drinking plenty of water, getting adequate sleep, and managing stress. These habits can support weight management and overall well-being.

- **Professional Guidance:** Consider seeking guidance from a healthcare provider, nutritionist, or fitness professional to develop a personalized plan that aligns with your health goals. Professional support can provide you with tailored advice and help you overcome challenges.

By adopting a balanced diet, engaging in regular exercise, and making gradual, sustainable changes, you can achieve and maintain a healthy weight, improving your HRV. Monitoring your weight and staying committed to healthy habits will support your overall well-being and enhance your autonomic nervous system function.

Smoking and Alcohol Consumption

Both smoking and excessive alcohol consumption can significantly lower HRV. Understanding how these habits affect your HRV and taking steps to quit smoking and moderate alcohol intake can lead to noticeable improvements in your overall health and autonomic function.

Impact of Smoking on HRV

Smoking introduces harmful chemicals into the body, including nicotine and carbon monoxide, which adversely affect cardiovascular function and reduce HRV. Nicotine stimulates the sympathetic nervous system, causing an increase in heart rate and blood pressure while lowering HRV. Long-term smoking leads to chronic inflammation, oxidative stress, and damage to blood vessels, further impairing autonomic balance.

Quitting Smoking

- **Health Benefits:** Quitting smoking can significantly improve cardiovascular health, lung function, and overall well-being. Within weeks of quitting, you may notice improvements in HRV as your autonomic nervous system begins to recover.

- **Support and Resources:** Seek support from healthcare professionals, smoking cessation programs, and support groups. Nicotine replacement therapy, prescription medications, and counseling can also aid in quitting.

- **Behavioral Strategies:** Adopt behavioral strategies to manage cravings and avoid triggers. Exercise, practice stress-reducing techniques, and stay connected with supportive friends and family.

Impact of Alcohol Consumption on HRV

Alcohol, particularly when consumed in large quantities, disrupts autonomic balance and lowers HRV. Acute alcohol consumption can temporarily reduce HRV by increasing sympathetic activity and decreasing parasympathetic activity. Chronic heavy drinking leads to long-term autonomic dysfunction, liver damage, and increased risk of cardiovascular diseases, further lowering HRV.

Moderating Alcohol Intake

- **Health Benefits:** Moderating alcohol intake or abstaining from alcohol can improve HRV, liver function, and overall health. Reduced alcohol consumption lowers the risk of hypertension, heart disease, and other alcohol-related health issues.

- **Guidelines:** Follow recommended guidelines for alcohol consumption, which suggest limiting intake to moderate levels—up to one drink per day for women and up to two drinks per day for men.

- **Alternative Activities:** Find alternative activities that do not involve alcohol. Engage in hobbies, exercise, and social activities that promote well-being without the adverse effects of alcohol.

- **Support and Resources:** If you find it challenging to moderate your alcohol intake, seek support from healthcare professionals, counseling services, and support groups like Alcoholics Anonymous (AA).

Combined Effects and Lifestyle Changes

The combined effects of smoking and excessive alcohol consumption can exacerbate their negative impact on HRV and overall health. Addressing both habits simultaneously can lead to more significant health improvements and better HRV outcomes.

- **Holistic Approach:** Adopt a holistic approach to health by combining efforts to quit smoking and moderate alcohol intake with other healthy lifestyle changes. Focus on a balanced diet, regular exercise, stress management, and good sleep hygiene to support overall well-being.

- **Regular Monitoring:** Monitor your HRV regularly to track improvements as you make these lifestyle changes. Use HRV data to stay motivated and adjust your strategies as needed.

By quitting smoking and moderating alcohol intake, you can significantly improve your HRV and enhance your overall health. Seek support and use available resources to make these positive changes, as they are crucial for maintaining a healthy autonomic nervous system and improving your quality of life.

Environmental Factors

Environmental factors like air quality, temperature, and noise can influence HRV. Poor air quality and pollutant exposure can lower HRV by increasing bodily stress. Similarly, extreme temperatures and loud noises can disrupt autonomic function. Creating a healthy living environment can positively impact your HRV.

Air Quality

Poor air quality, including exposure to particulate matter, carbon monoxide, and volatile organic compounds (VOCs), can significantly reduce HRV. Inhalation of these pollutants can cause oxidative stress, inflammation, and respiratory issues, negatively affecting autonomic function.

Improving Air Quality

- **Ventilation:** Ensure your living space is well-ventilated to reduce the concentration of indoor pollutants. Use exhaust fans and open windows, and consider using air purifiers with HEPA filters to improve air quality.

- **Indoor Plants:** Certain indoor plants can help improve air quality by absorbing pollutants and releasing oxygen. Plants like spider plants, peace lilies, and snake plants are known for their air-purifying properties.

- **Avoid Smoking Indoors:** Smoking indoors releases harmful chemicals into the air, affecting both your HRV and the health of others in your household. If you smoke, do so outside and away from windows and doors.

Temperature

Extreme temperatures, whether too hot or cold, can stress the body and disrupt autonomic function, leading to lower HRV. Maintaining a comfortable and stable temperature in your living environment can support better HRV.

Maintaining Comfortable Temperature

- **Heating and Cooling Systems:** Use heating and cooling systems to maintain a comfortable indoor temperature. The ideal indoor temperature for most people is between 60-67°F (15-19°C) for sleeping and around 68-72°F (20-22°C) during the day.

- **Insulation:** Proper insulation can help maintain a stable indoor temperature, reducing the need for excessive heating or cooling.

- **Layering Clothing:** Dress in layers to quickly adjust to temperature changes and maintain comfort.

Noise

Loud and constant background noise can disrupt autonomic function and lower HRV by increasing stress levels. Creating a quieter living environment can help improve HRV.

Reducing Noise Pollution:

- **Soundproofing:** Use soundproofing materials like heavy curtains, carpets, and acoustic panels to reduce noise levels in your home.

- **White Noise Machines:** Consider using white noise machines or apps to mask disruptive sounds, especially during sleep.

- **Quiet Hours:** Establish quiet hours in your household, especially during nighttime, to ensure a peaceful environment for rest.

Light Exposure

Light exposure, particularly artificial light at night, can affect your circadian rhythm and HRV. Exposure to blue light from screens can disrupt melatonin production and sleep quality, impacting your autonomic balance.

Managing Light Exposure:

- **Natural Light:** Maximize exposure to natural light during the day to support your circadian rhythm.

- **Dim Lights in the Evening:** Use dim lighting in the evening to signal to your body that it's time to wind down. Avoid bright screens and use blue light filters on electronic devices.

- **Dark Sleep Environment:** Use blackout curtains or a sleep mask to ensure your bedroom is dark during sleep.

Creating a Healthy Living Environment

By making small changes to improve air quality, maintain comfortable temperatures, reduce noise pollution, and manage light exposure, you can create a healthier living environment that supports optimal HRV. Regularly assess your environment and adjust to promote well-being and autonomic balance.

Breathing Patterns

Breathing patterns have a direct impact on HRV. Deep, slow breathing activates the parasympathetic nervous system, increasing HRV. Controlled breathing exercises like diaphragmatic or box breathing can help improve your HRV. Incorporate these techniques into your daily routine, especially during stressful moments, to enhance your autonomic balance and overall well-being.

The Impact of Breathing Patterns on HRV

Breathing directly influences the autonomic nervous system. Rapid, shallow breathing tends to activate the sympathetic nervous system, which can decrease HRV. Conversely, deep, slow breathing stimulates the parasympathetic nervous system, promoting relaxation and increasing HRV. You can enhance your autonomic balance and improve HRV by consciously adjusting your breathing patterns.

Diaphragmatic Breathing

Diaphragmatic breathing, also known as belly breathing, involves breathing deeply into the diaphragm rather than shallowly into the chest. This technique helps activate the parasympathetic nervous system and increase HRV.

How to Practice Diaphragmatic Breathing:

- **Find a Comfortable Position:** Sit or lie down in a comfortable position.

- **Place Your Hands:** Place one hand on your chest and the other on your abdomen.

- **Inhale Deeply:** Take a slow, deep breath in through your nose, allowing your abdomen to rise while keeping your chest relatively still.

- **Exhale Slowly:** Exhale slowly through your mouth, feeling your abdomen fall.

- **Repeat:** Continue this pattern for 5-10 minutes, focusing on deep, rhythmic breaths.

Box Breathing

Box breathing, or square breathing, is a simple technique involving breathing in a four-step pattern. This method is effective for reducing stress and enhancing HRV.

How to Practice Box Breathing:

- **Inhale:** Breathe deeply through your nose for a count of four.

- **Hold:** Hold your breath for a count of four.

- **Exhale:** Exhale slowly through your mouth for a count of four.

- **Hold:** Hold your breath again for a count of four.

- **Repeat:** Continue this cycle for several minutes, maintaining a steady, even rhythm.

Incorporating Breathing Exercises into Your Routine

Regular controlled breathing exercises can significantly improve your HRV and overall well-being. Here are some tips for integrating these techniques into your daily life:

- **Daily Practice:** Set aside time each day for dedicated breathing practice. Even just 5-10 minutes can make a difference.

- **During Stressful Moments:** Use deep, slow breathing to calm yourself during stressful situations. This can help prevent sympathetic nervous system activation and maintain higher HRV.

- **Before Bed:** Practice diaphragmatic or box breathing before bedtime to promote relaxation and improve sleep quality.

- **Mindfulness Integration:** Combine breathing exercises with mindfulness meditation to enhance the benefits. Focus on your breath and stay present in the moment to further reduce stress and improve HRV.

Incorporating controlled breathing exercises into your daily routine can enhance your autonomic balance, increase your HRV, and improve your overall health and well-being. These simple, effective techniques are powerful tools for managing stress and supporting cardiovascular health.

Social Interactions

Positive social interactions and strong relationships can boost HRV. Engaging in meaningful conversations, spending time with loved ones, and participating in social activities can enhance your mood and reduce stress. On the other hand, negative social interactions and isolation can lower HRV. Prioritize building healthy relationships to support your HRV and overall mental health.

Impact of Positive Social Interactions on HRV

Positive social interactions activate the parasympathetic nervous system, promoting relaxation and increasing HRV. Here's how social connections can improve HRV:

- **Emotional Support:** A robust support system provides emotional support during stressful times. Knowing you have people who care about you and are there for you can reduce stress and enhance your autonomic balance.

- **Sense of Belonging:** Being part of a community or group gives you a sense of belonging and purpose. This can boost your mood and reduce feelings of loneliness and anxiety, which positively affects HRV.

- **Laughter and Joy:** Sharing joyful moments and laughter with others releases endorphins and reduces stress hormones, leading to higher HRV. Laughter therapy and social activities that induce laughter can significantly benefit your heart health.

Building and Maintaining Healthy Relationships

Building and maintaining healthy relationships requires effort and intention. Here are some tips to foster positive social interactions:

- **Quality Time:** Spend quality time with friends and family. Engage in activities you enjoy together, have meaningful conversations, and be present in the moment. Regular social interactions strengthen bonds and enhance your emotional well-being.

- **Active Listening:** Practice active listening when interacting with others. Show genuine interest in what they say, provide empathetic responses, and avoid interrupting. Active listening fosters deeper connections and builds trust.

- **Social Activities:** Participate in social activities and community events. Join clubs, volunteer organizations, or hobby groups where you can meet new people and build meaningful relationships. Social engagement promotes a sense of belonging and community.

- **Expressing Gratitude:** Express gratitude and appreciation to those around you. Acknowledge their positive impact on your life and show appreciation for their support. Gratitude strengthens relationships and enhances emotional bonds.

Avoiding Negative Social Interactions

While positive social interactions boost HRV, negative social interactions and isolation can have the opposite effect. Here's how to manage negative social influences:

- **Set Boundaries:** Set healthy boundaries with individuals who may cause stress or negativity in your life. Protecting your emotional well-being is crucial for maintaining high HRV.

- **Conflict Resolution:** Learn practical conflict resolution skills to handle disagreements constructively. Address conflicts calmly and respectfully, and seek to find mutually beneficial solutions.

- **Social Media Management:** Be mindful of your social media usage. While it can be a tool for staying connected, excessive use or negative interactions on social media can increase stress and lower HRV. Limit your screen time and curate your feed to include positive content.

Combating Social Isolation

Social isolation can significantly lower HRV and negatively impact mental health. To combat isolation:

- **Reach Out:** If you feel isolated, contact friends, family, or support groups. Initiate conversations and make plans to connect with others.

- **Join Support Groups:** Consider joining support groups or therapy groups where you can share experiences and receive emotional support from others facing similar challenges.

- **Stay Connected:** Use technology to stay connected with loved ones, especially if you cannot meet in person. Video calls, phone calls, and messaging apps can help bridge the gap and maintain social connections.

By prioritizing positive social interactions and building solid relationships, you can improve your HRV and overall mental health. Engaging with others in meaningful ways supports your emotional well-being and enhances your autonomic function, leading to a healthier and more fulfilling life.

Mindfulness and Meditation

Mindfulness and meditation practices are powerful tools for improving HRV. These practices promote relaxation and reduce stress, leading to higher HRV. Regular mindfulness sessions can profoundly impact your autonomic function, whether through guided meditations, yoga, or simply being present in the moment. Here's how to incorporate mindfulness into your daily routine to experience its benefits on your HRV.

Understanding Mindfulness and Meditation

Mindfulness is being fully present and engaged in the current moment without judgment. It involves paying attention to your thoughts, feelings, and sensations as they arise, fostering a sense of awareness and acceptance.

Meditation is a broader practice encompassing various techniques aimed at focusing the mind and achieving a state of calm and clarity.

Typical forms of meditation include mindfulness, loving-kindness, and transcendental meditation.

Benefits of Mindfulness and Meditation on HRV

Regular mindfulness and meditation have increased HRV by promoting parasympathetic nervous system activity and reducing sympathetic dominance. Here are some key benefits:

- **Stress Reduction:** Mindfulness and meditation help reduce stress by calming the mind and lowering cortisol levels, the stress hormone. Reduced stress levels lead to higher HRV and better overall autonomic balance.

- **Improved Emotional Regulation:** These practices enhance your ability to manage emotions, reducing the impact of negative emotions on your heart rate and autonomic function. Improved emotional regulation supports higher HRV.

- **Enhanced Relaxation:** Meditation and mindfulness promote relaxation, which increases parasympathetic activity and boosts HRV. The relaxation response counteracts the effects of chronic stress and sympathetic overactivity.

Incorporating Mindfulness and Meditation into Your Routine

- **Daily Practice:** Set aside time each day for mindfulness or meditation practice. Even just 5-10 minutes a day can make a significant difference. Gradually increase the duration as you become more comfortable with the practice.

- **Guided Meditations:** Use guided meditation apps or videos to help you get started. These resources provide structured sessions that can guide you through various meditation techniques.

- **Mindful Breathing:** Practice mindful breathing by focusing on your breath and paying attention to each inhale and exhale. This simple practice can be done anytime and anywhere to help you stay grounded and present.

- **Yoga:** Incorporate yoga into your routine to combine physical movement with mindfulness and deep breathing. Yoga enhances flexibility, strength, and relaxation, contributing to higher HRV.

- **Mindfulness in Daily Activities:** Practice mindfulness during everyday activities, such as eating, walking, or washing dishes. Focus on the sensations, sights, and sounds around you, and engage fully in the present moment.

Tips for Successful Practice

- **Find a Quiet Space:** Choose a quiet, comfortable space to practice without distractions. Create a calming environment with soft lighting and minimal noise.

- **Consistency:** Consistency is crucial in reaping the benefits of mindfulness and meditation. Aim to practice at the same time each day to establish a routine.

- **Be Patient:** Be patient with yourself as you develop your practice. It's normal for the mind to wander; gently bring your focus back to the present moment without judgment.

- **Stay Open-Minded:** Approach mindfulness and meditation with an open mind. Experiment with different techniques to find what works best for you.

Incorporating mindfulness and meditation into your daily routine can enhance your autonomic function, increase HRV, and improve your overall well-being. These practices offer a robust, accessible way to manage stress and support cardiovascular health.

Time of Day

HRV can vary throughout the day and is influenced by your circadian rhythm and daily activities. Generally, HRV is higher in the morning and gradually decreases as the day progresses. To get the most accurate readings, measure your HRV at the same time each day, preferably in the morning. Understanding your daily HRV patterns can help you make informed decisions about your activities and optimize your health strategies.

The Influence of Circadian Rhythm on HRV

The circadian rhythm is your body's internal clock, regulating various physiological processes over a 24-hour cycle. This rhythm affects your autonomic nervous system and, consequently, your HRV. In the morning, after a night of rest, your parasympathetic activity is typically higher, resulting in increased HRV. As the day progresses and you engage in various activities, sympathetic activity rises, gradually decreasing HRV.

Measuring HRV at the Same Time Each Day

To obtain consistent and accurate HRV readings, it's essential to measure your HRV at the same time each day. Morning measurements are ideal because they provide a baseline less affected by the stresses and activities of daily life. Here are some tips for measuring your HRV:

- **Morning Routine:** Incorporate HRV measurement into your morning routine. Measure your HRV shortly after waking up, ideally before engaging in physical activities or consuming food or beverages (except water).

- **Consistency:** Use the same device and follow the same measurement protocol daily to ensure consistency.

- **Environment:** Measure HRV in a calm, quiet environment to minimize external influences affecting your readings.

Understanding Daily HRV Patterns

Recognizing how your HRV fluctuates throughout the day can help you better understand your body's responses to different activities and stressors. Tracking your HRV over time allows you to identify patterns and make informed decisions to optimize your health and well-being. Here are some key points to consider:

- **Morning Readings:** Higher HRV readings suggest good recovery and autonomic balance. Use these readings as your baseline.

- **Daily Activities:** Monitor how different activities (e.g., exercise, work, meals) impact your HRV. Activities that significantly lower your HRV may indicate higher stress or physical exertion.

- **Evening Readings:** Lower HRV in the evening is expected, reflecting the cumulative effects of the day's activities. However, consistently low evening HRV may indicate chronic stress or inadequate recovery.

Using HRV Patterns to Optimize Health Strategies

By understanding your daily HRV patterns, you can better decide your activities and health strategies. Here's how:

- **Exercise Timing:** Schedule high-intensity workouts when your HRV is higher (e.g., late morning or early afternoon) to optimize performance and recovery.

- **Stress Management:** Identify periods of low HRV and incorporate stress-reducing activities (e.g., mindfulness, meditation, or light exercise) to support autonomic balance.

- **Recovery Monitoring:** Use morning HRV readings to assess your recovery from previous activities. Adjust your routine if your HRV remains consistently low in the morning, indicating inadequate recovery.

Practical Tips for Daily HRV Measurement

- **Routine:** Establish a consistent routine for HRV measurement, making it a part of your daily habit.

- **Documentation:** Keep a log of your HRV readings and notes on your activities, sleep quality, and stress levels. This will help you identify patterns and correlations.

- **Adjustments:** Be flexible and adjust your routine based on your HRV data. This proactive approach can help you maintain optimal autonomic balance and overall health.

By measuring your HRV at the same time each day and understanding your daily HRV patterns, you can make informed decisions about your activities and health strategies. Consistent monitoring and analysis of HRV data can provide valuable insights into your body's responses, helping you optimize your well-being and performance.

Caffeine and Stimulants

Caffeine and other stimulants can temporarily lower HRV by increasing sympathetic nervous system activity. While moderate caffeine consumption is generally safe, excessive intake can negatively impact your HRV. Here's how to monitor and manage caffeine intake to support your autonomic balance and improve your HRV.

Impact of Caffeine on HRV

Caffeine is a central nervous system stimulant that can increase alertness and energy levels. However, it also stimulates the release of adrenaline, activating the sympathetic nervous system and temporarily lowering HRV. The effects of caffeine can vary depending on individual sensitivity, the amount consumed, and the time of day it is consumed.

Moderate Caffeine Consumption

Moderate caffeine consumption is generally considered safe for most people. The key is to balance the stimulating effects of caffeine with the need to maintain autonomic balance. Here are some guidelines for moderate caffeine consumption:

- **Daily Limit:** Aim to limit your caffeine intake to 200-400 mg per day (about 2-4 cups of coffee). This amount is typically safe for most adults and unlikely to cause significant disruptions to HRV.

- **Timing:** Avoid consuming caffeine late afternoon or evening, as it can interfere with sleep and recovery, leading to lower HRV. Morning or early afternoon consumption is preferable.

- **Monitor Effects:** Pay attention to how your body responds to caffeine. If you notice significant drops in HRV or increased feelings of stress and anxiety, consider reducing your intake.

Managing Excessive Caffeine Intake

Excessive caffeine consumption can negatively affect HRV, sleep quality, and overall health. Here are some strategies to manage and reduce excessive caffeine intake:

- **Gradual Reduction:** If you consume a high amount of caffeine, reduce your intake gradually to avoid withdrawal symptoms such as headaches, irritability, and fatigue. Cut back by one cup daily until you reach a more moderate level.

- **Healthy Alternatives:** Replace caffeinated beverages with healthier alternatives, such as herbal teas, decaffeinated coffee, or water infused with fruits and herbs. These options can provide hydration and flavor without the stimulating effects of caffeine.

- **Mindful Consumption:** Be mindful of hidden sources of caffeine, such as energy drinks, certain soft drinks, and some medications. Read labels and choose products with lower or no caffeine content.

Opting for Healthier Alternatives

Switching to healthier alternatives can help support your autonomic balance and improve HRV. Here are some options to consider:

- **Herbal Teas:** Herbal teas, such as chamomile, peppermint, and rooibos, are naturally caffeine-free and can promote relaxation and hydration. Many herbal teas also have additional health benefits, such as aiding digestion and reducing stress.

- **Decaffeinated Beverages:** Decaffeinated coffee and tea provide the flavor and comfort of their caffeinated counterparts without the stimulating effects. Choose high-quality decaf options to enjoy your favorite beverages without impacting your HRV.

- **Water and Infused Water:** Staying well-hydrated is essential for maintaining good HRV. Infuse water with fruits, vegetables, or herbs (e.g., lemon, cucumber, mint) for a refreshing and hydrating alternative to caffeinated drinks.

Monitoring Your Caffeine Intake and HRV

Regularly monitor your HRV to observe how caffeine affects your autonomic function. Use this data to make informed decisions about your caffeine consumption. Here's how to do it:

- **Track HRV Trends:** Use an HRV monitoring device to track your HRV daily. Note any significant changes in your HRV readings related to your caffeine intake.

- **Adjust Intake:** If you notice high caffeine consumption correlates with lower HRV, consider reducing your intake and opting for healthier alternatives.

- **Consistency:** Maintain a consistent routine with moderate caffeine consumption to support stable HRV and overall well-being.

By monitoring your caffeine consumption and opting for healthier alternatives, you can support your autonomic balance and improve your HRV. Moderate your intake to enjoy the benefits of caffeine without compromising your heart rate variability and overall health.

Nutrient Deficiencies

Nutrient deficiencies can affect HRV by disrupting overall bodily function. Ensuring a balanced diet of essential vitamins and minerals supports your autonomic nervous system and heart health. Pay particular attention to nutrients like magnesium, omega-3 fatty acids, and B vitamins, which are crucial in maintaining optimal HRV. If necessary, consider supplements to address specific deficiencies and improve your HRV.

Impact of Nutrient Deficiencies on HRV

Deficiencies in essential nutrients can impair the body's ability to maintain autonomic balance and cardiovascular health, leading to lower HRV. Here's how specific nutrients influence HRV:

Magnesium

Magnesium is vital for muscle and nerve function, including heart function. It helps regulate heart rhythm and promotes the relaxation of blood vessels, supporting better HRV. Magnesium deficiency can lead to increased stress and lower HRV.

Omega-3 Fatty Acids

Omega-3 fatty acids in fish and certain plant oils have anti-inflammatory properties and support heart health. They improve autonomic function by enhancing parasympathetic activity, which can lead to higher HRV. Low levels of omega-3s can contribute to increased cardiovascular risk and reduced HRV.

B Vitamins

B vitamins, especially B6, B12, and folate, are crucial for energy production, red blood cell formation, and neurological function. These vitamins help maintain healthy nerve function and reduce homocysteine levels associated with cardiovascular health. Deficiencies in B vitamins can impair autonomic regulation and lower HRV.

Ensuring a Balanced Diet

To support optimal HRV, focus on a balanced diet that includes a variety of nutrient-dense foods. Here are some tips:

- **Diverse Food Sources:** Incorporate a wide range of foods to ensure you get a broad spectrum of nutrients. Include plenty of fruits, vegetables, whole grains, lean proteins, nuts, seeds, and healthy fats.

- **Magnesium-Rich Foods:** Consume magnesium-rich foods, such as leafy green vegetables, nuts, seeds, whole grains, and legumes. Examples include spinach, almonds, pumpkin seeds, and black beans.

- **Omega-3 Fatty Acids:** Include sources of omega-3 fatty acids in your diet, such as fatty fish (salmon, mackerel, sardines), flaxseeds, chia seeds, and walnuts. If you don't consume enough through diet, consider taking a high-quality fish oil supplement.

- **B Vitamins:** Eat foods rich in B vitamins, such as whole grains, eggs, dairy products, meat (especially liver), legumes, and leafy green vegetables. Fortified cereals and nutritional yeast can also be good sources.

Considering Supplements

If you struggle to get enough of these nutrients through diet alone, supplements can help address specific deficiencies. Here's how to approach supplementation:

- **Consult with a Healthcare Provider:** Before starting any supplements, consult your healthcare provider to identify your specific needs and avoid potential interactions with other medications.

- **Magnesium Supplements:** Consider magnesium supplements if you have difficulty meeting your needs through diet.

Magnesium citrate and magnesium glycinate are well-absorbed forms.

- **Omega-3 Supplements:** Fish oil supplements can provide a convenient source of omega-3 fatty acids. Choose high-quality, purified options for products that contain both EPA and DHA.

- **B Vitamin Supplements:** B complex supplements can ensure a balanced intake of essential B vitamins. Look for methylated forms of B12 (methylcobalamin) and folate (methylfolate) for better absorption.

Monitoring and Adjusting

Regularly monitor your nutrient intake and HRV to identify any correlations. Adjust your diet and supplementation to support optimal HRV and overall health. Here's how:

- **Track Your Intake:** Keep a food diary or use a nutrition tracking app to monitor your intake of essential nutrients. This can help you identify any gaps in your diet.

- **Measure HRV:** Use an HRV monitoring device to track your HRV regularly. Note any changes in your readings with dietary adjustments and supplementation.

- **Adjust Accordingly:** Adjust your diet and supplementation based on your HRV data and nutrient intake. Continuously fine-tune your approach to achieve the best outcomes for your autonomic function and heart health.

By ensuring a balanced diet rich in essential vitamins and minerals and considering supplements when necessary, you can support your autonomic nervous system and improve your HRV. Addressing nutrient deficiencies is critical to maintaining overall health and optimizing heart rate variability.

Posture

Your posture can influence HRV by affecting your breathing patterns and overall comfort. Poor posture can lead to shallow breathing and increased bodily stress, lowering HRV. Practicing good posture by keeping your spine aligned, your shoulders relaxed, and your breathing deeply can support better HRV and overall health. Here's how to maintain proper posture and its benefits for HRV.

The Impact of Posture on HRV

Breathing Patterns

Poor posture, such as slouching or hunching over, can compress your diaphragm and restrict your lungs' ability to expand fully. This leads to shallow breathing, which limits oxygen intake and increases sympathetic nervous system activity, reducing HRV.

Musculoskeletal Stress

Bad posture unnecessarily strains your muscles, ligaments, and joints. This chronic stress can trigger pain and discomfort, activating the body's stress response and lowering HRV.

Practicing Good Posture

Sitting Posture

When sitting, especially for long periods, follow these guidelines to maintain good posture:

- **Spine Alignment:** Keep your back straight and aligned with your spine's natural curves. Avoid slumping or leaning forward.

- **Feet Position:** Place your feet flat on the floor, with knees at a right angle and hips level with or slightly higher than your knees.

- **Chair Support:** Use a chair that supports your lower back. Place a small cushion or rolled towel behind your lower back for extra support if necessary.

- **Shoulder Position:** Keep your shoulders relaxed and slightly pulled back. Avoid rounding your shoulders forward.

- **Head Position:** Ensure your head is aligned with your spine, with your chin slightly tucked to avoid forward head posture.

Standing Posture

When standing, practice the following to maintain good posture:

- **Feet Position:** Stand with your feet shoulder-width apart and distribute your weight evenly on both feet.

- **Knee Position:** Keep your knees slightly bent, not locked.

- **Pelvis Position:** Tuck your pelvis slightly to engage your core muscles and support your lower back.

- **Spine Alignment:** Maintain the natural curves of your spine, avoiding excessive arching or rounding.

- **Shoulder and Head Position:** Keep your shoulders relaxed and pulled back, with your head aligned over your spine.

Checking and Correcting Posture

Regular Self-Check

Regularly check your posture throughout the day, especially if you have a sedentary job. Set reminders to assess and correct your posture every hour. Use mirrors or the reflection in your monitor to help you align your posture correctly.

Ergonomic Workspace

Ensure your workspace is ergonomically designed to support good posture. Adjust your chair, desk, and monitor height so your screen is at eye level and your keyboard and mouse are within easy reach without straining.

Stretching and Mobility Exercises

Incorporate stretching and mobility exercises into your daily routine to counteract the effects of prolonged sitting and improve your posture. Focus on stretches that open the chest, shoulders, and hips and strengthen your core and back muscles.

Benefits of Good Posture for HRV

Improved Breathing

Maintaining good posture allows your diaphragm to function optimally, promoting deep, diaphragmatic breathing. This enhances oxygen intake and activates the parasympathetic nervous system, increasing HRV.

Reduced Stress and Pain

Good posture minimizes musculoskeletal strain, reducing discomfort and pain. This helps lower overall bodily stress and supports better autonomic balance, improving HRV.

Enhanced Comfort and Productivity

Good posture enhances overall comfort and can improve productivity, especially in sedentary work environments. A comfortable and pain-free body is less likely to trigger stress responses, supporting higher HRV.

Good posture can improve your breathing patterns, reduce bodily stress, and enhance your HRV. Regularly check and correct your posture, incorporate ergonomic adjustments, and engage in stretching exercises to support better overall health and well-being.

Marijuana

Marijuana use can have varying effects on HRV, depending on the individual and the frequency of use. While some studies suggest that marijuana can increase HRV by promoting relaxation, others indicate potential adverse impacts, particularly with chronic use. Understanding how marijuana affects your HRV and making informed decisions based on your readings is essential for maintaining overall health and well-being.

The Effects of Marijuana on HRV

Promoting Relaxation

Some research indicates that marijuana can increase HRV by promoting relaxation and reducing stress. The active compounds in marijuana, mainly THC (tetrahydrocannabinol) and CBD (cannabidiol) can activate the parasympathetic nervous system, leading to higher HRV.

Potential Negative Impacts

Chronic or heavy marijuana use, however, can lead to adverse effects on HRV. Regular use may cause changes in the autonomic nervous system, reducing HRV over time. Additionally, smoking marijuana can introduce harmful substances into the lungs, impacting cardiovascular and respiratory health.

Individual Variability

The effects of marijuana on HRV can vary significantly from person to person. Factors such as genetics, overall health, tolerance, and the specific strain or form of marijuana used can influence how HRV is affected. It is essential to monitor your response to marijuana and adjust your usage accordingly.

Monitoring Marijuana's Impact on HRV

Regular HRV Measurement

Use an HRV monitoring device to track your HRV regularly, especially when using marijuana. To identify patterns, note any changes in your HRV readings before and after use.

Personalized Data

Pay attention to how different strains, dosages, and methods of consumption (e.g., smoking, vaping, edibles) affect your HRV. Use this personalized data to make informed decisions about your marijuana use.

Moderation and Mindfulness

Moderate Use

If you choose to use marijuana, moderation is key. Occasional use may promote relaxation without significantly impacting HRV, while chronic or heavy use may have adverse effects. Balance marijuana use with other healthy lifestyle practices.

Mindful Consumption

Be cognizant of when and how you use marijuana. Avoid using it as a primary coping mechanism for stress or anxiety, as this can lead to dependency. Instead, incorporate other stress management techniques such as exercise, meditation, and social interactions.

Making Informed Decisions

Consult with Healthcare Providers

If you use marijuana regularly or have concerns about its impact on your HRV and overall health, consult with a healthcare provider. They can provide guidance tailored to your individual health needs and help you make informed decisions.

Balanced Lifestyle

Ensure that your marijuana use does not interfere with maintaining a balanced lifestyle. Prioritize a healthy diet, regular exercise, adequate sleep, and strong social connections to support your HRV and overall well-being.

Potential Benefits and Risks

Potential Benefits

For some individuals, marijuana may offer therapeutic benefits such as pain relief, improved sleep, and reduced anxiety, which can indirectly support better HRV. CBD, in particular, is often used for its calming effects without the psychoactive properties of THC.

Potential Risks

Be aware of possible risks, including impaired cognitive function, dependency, and respiratory issues associated with smoking. Monitor your health closely and adjust to minimize these risks.

By monitoring how marijuana affects your HRV and using it mindfully and in moderation, you can ensure that any substance use supports your overall health and well-being. Personalized data and informed decisions are crucial to maintaining optimal HRV and a balanced lifestyle.

Understanding and managing these various habits and factors can significantly influence your HRV and optimize your health. In the next chapter, we'll explore how to create a personalized HRV improvement plan, helping you take actionable steps toward enhancing your well-being based on your HRV data.

Chapter Four

Creating Your HRV Improvement Plan

With your HRV data and the knowledge you've acquired, we'll guide you in creating a personalized plan to improve your HRV. You'll explore lifestyle changes, nutritional adjustments, and exercise strategies to enhance your HRV.

Assessing Your Current HRV Status

Before embarking on a journey to improve your HRV, it's crucial to establish a clear understanding of your current status. Start by consistently measuring your HRV over some time—ideally, a few weeks. Use a reliable HRV monitoring device and take measurements at the same time each day, preferably in the morning. This consistency will provide an accurate baseline, reflecting your autonomic nervous system's current state.

Take note of any patterns or trends in your HRV data. Do specific days or activities correlate with higher or lower HRV readings?

Understanding these correlations will help you identify factors that positively or negatively impact your HRV. Keep a journal of your daily activities, diet, sleep quality, stress levels, and any significant events. This comprehensive record will be valuable as you implement changes to improve your HRV.

Setting Goals and Tracking Progress

With a clear picture of your current HRV status, the next step is to set achievable goals. These goals should be specific, measurable, attainable, relevant, and time-bound (SMART). For example, instead of setting a vague goal like "improve my HRV," aim for something more concrete, such as "increase my average morning HRV by 10% over the next three months."

Break down your main goal into smaller, actionable steps. For instance, if improving sleep quality is part of your plan, specific actions might include establishing a consistent bedtime routine, reducing screen time before bed, and creating a sleep-friendly environment. Similarly, if stress management is a focus, incorporate daily mindfulness practices, regular physical activity, and time for relaxation into your schedule.

Track your progress by regularly reviewing your HRV data and comparing it to your baseline. Use apps or software that sync with your HRV monitor to visualize your data over time. Celebrate small victories along the way to stay motivated. Adjust your plan based on your progress and any new insights you gain about factors affecting your HRV.

Implementing Lifestyle Changes

Improving HRV is often about making small, consistent changes across various aspects of your lifestyle. Here are some key areas to focus on:

- **Stress Management**: Incorporate techniques like meditation, deep breathing exercises, yoga, and other relaxation practices into your daily routine. Prioritize activities that help you unwind and manage stress effectively.

- **Diet**: Aim for a balanced diet rich in whole foods, including plenty of fruits, vegetables, lean proteins, and healthy fats. Avoid processed foods, excessive sugars, and unhealthy fats. Pay attention to how different foods affect your HRV and adjust your diet accordingly.

- **Physical Activity**: Maintain a regular exercise routine, including aerobic and anaerobic activities. Ensure you're not overtraining by including rest days and varying the intensity of your workouts. Listen to your body and adjust your training based on your HRV trends.

- **Sleep Quality**: Prioritize sleeping 7-9 hours each night. Establish a consistent sleep schedule, create a comfortable environment, and develop a relaxing pre-bedtime routine to improve sleep quality.

- **Hydration**: Stay well-hydrated by drinking sufficient water throughout the day. Monitor your fluid intake and ensure you're replenishing fluids lost during exercise.

- **Mindfulness and Meditation**: Regular mindfulness and meditation practices can significantly enhance your HRV by promoting relaxation and reducing stress. Incorporate these practices into your daily routine, even just for a few minutes each day.

Monitoring and Adjusting Your Plan

Regularly review your HRV data to assess the effectiveness of your improvement plan. Pay attention to trends and patterns, and adjust your strategies as needed. If you notice a consistent increase in your HRV, it's a sign that your efforts are paying off. However, if your HRV remains stagnant or declines, it may be time to reevaluate your approach.

Consider seeking support from a healthcare professional or a coach specializing in HRV and lifestyle optimization. They can provide personalized guidance and help you fine-tune your plan to achieve better results.

Long-Term Commitment to HRV Improvement

Improving HRV is not a one-time effort but a long-term commitment to a healthier lifestyle. Consistency and perseverance are key. You can maintain and enhance your autonomic balance over time by continuously monitoring your HRV and making informed adjustments to your habits.

Remember, the goal is to achieve higher HRV and improve your overall well-being. By focusing on holistic health practices and making sustainable lifestyle changes, you'll enhance your HRV and enjoy a better quality of life.

Conclusion

As we reach the end of *Heart Rate Variability Essentials: Discover How Your Habits Shape This Vital Biomarker*, I hope you've gained valuable insights into how HRV can be a powerful tool for enhancing your health and well-being. By understanding the basics of HRV, learning how to monitor it effectively, and implementing strategies to improve it, you are now equipped to make informed decisions about your lifestyle and health practices.

Remember, the journey to optimal health is a continuous process. Regularly assess your HRV, make adjustments based on your findings, and stay committed to the healthy habits you've learned. Whether through better stress management, a balanced diet, regular physical activity, or quality sleep, each step brings you closer to achieving and maintaining a higher HRV and, consequently, a healthier life.

I encourage you to keep exploring and experimenting with different strategies to see what works best for you. Stay curious, stay motivated, and don't hesitate to seek professional guidance if needed. Your commitment to improving your HRV is a testament to your dedication to a healthier, more vibrant life.

Finally, I have a small request. If you found this book helpful, please consider leaving a review on Amazon. Your feedback helps other readers discover the benefits of HRV and supports me in my mission to provide valuable health information. Your review can make a significant difference.

Thank you for joining me on this journey to better health through HRV optimization. Here's to your continued success and well-being!

References

1. Allen, A. P., Kennedy, P. J., Cryan, J. F., Dinan, T. G., & Clarke, G. (2014). Biological and psychological markers of stress in humans: Focus on the Trier Social Stress Test. Neuroscience & Biobehavioral Reviews, 38, 94-124. https://www.sciencedirect.com/science/article/pii/S014976341300274X

2. Black, D. S., & Slavich, G. M. (2016). Mindfulness meditation and the immune system: A systematic review of randomized controlled trials. Annals of the New York Academy of Sciences, 1373(1), 13-24. https://nyaspubs.onlinelibrary.wiley.com/doi/full/10.1111/nyas.12998

3. Borresen, J., & Lambert, M. I. (2009). The quantification of training load, the training response and the effect on performance. Sports Medicine, 39(9), 779-795. https://link.springer.com/article/10.2165/11317780-000000000-00000

4. Calder, P. C. (2013). Omega-3 polyunsaturated fatty acids and inflammatory processes: Nutrition or pharmacology? British Journal of Clinical Pharmacology, 75(3),

645-662. https://bpspubs.onlinelibrary.wiley.com/doi/full/10.1111/j.1365-2125.2010.03727.x

5. Calder, P. C., Ahluwalia, N., Brouns, F., Buetler, T., Clement, K., Cunningham, K., ... & Serra-Majem, L. (2011). Dietary factors and low-grade inflammation in relation to overweight and obesity. British Journal of Nutrition, 106(S3), S5-S78. https://www.cambridge.org/core/journals/british-journal-of-nutrition/article/dietary-factors-and-lowgrade-inflammation-in-relation-to-overweight-and-obesity/6CF06D53B6BC4916E6BDE8A7EAC2D2B8

6. Dempsey, P. C., Mathiassen, S. E., Jackson, J. A., & Potter, K. M. (2015). Sitting posture and sedentary exposure duration: Analysis of objective exposure variability and subjectively reported health in call centre workers. International Journal of Industrial Ergonomics, 48, 113-121. https://www.sciencedirect.com/science/article/abs/pii/S0169814115000845

7. Goyal, M., Singh, S., Sibinga, E. M. S., Gould, N. F., Rowland Seymour, A., Sharma, R., ... & Haythornthwaite, J. A. (2014). Meditation programs for psychological stress and well-being: A systematic review and meta-analysis. JAMA Internal Medicine, 174(3), 357-368. https://jamanetwork.com/journals/jamainternalmedicine/fullarticle/1809754

8. Grandner, M. A., & Kripke, D. F. (2004). Self-reported sleep complaints with long-term use of hypnotics in a general population sample. Psychiatry and Clinical Neurosciences, 58(6), 651-657. https://onlinelibrary.wiley.com/doi/abs/1

0.1111/j.1440-1819.2004.01236.x

9. Gruber, S. A., Silveri, M. M., Dahlgren, M. K., & Yurgelun-Todd, D. (2011). Why so impulsive? White matter alterations are associated with impulsivity in chronic marijuana smokers. Experimental and Clinical Psychopharmacology, 19(3), 231-242. https://psycnet.apa.org/doi/10.1037/a0023366

10. Harris, W. S., & Mozaffarian, D. (2008). Omega-3 fatty acids and cardiovascular disease: Evidence explained and mechanisms explored. Clinical Lipidology, 3(1), 25-38. https://www.futuremedicine.com/doi/abs/10.2217/17460898.3.1.25

11. Hirshkowitz, M., Whiton, K., Albert, S. M., Alessi, C., Bruni, O., DonCarlos, L., ... & Adams Hillard, P. J. (2015). National Sleep Foundation's sleep time duration recommendations: Methodology and results summary. Sleep Health, 1(1), 40-43. https://www.sleephealthjournal.org/article/S2352-7218(15)00015-7/fulltext

12. Holt-Lunstad, J., Smith, T. B., & Layton, J. B. (2010). Social relationships and mortality risk: A meta-analytic review. PLOS Medicine, 7(7), e1000316. https://journals.plos.org/plosmedicine/article?id=10.1371/journal.pmed.1000316

13. Jarvis, M. J., Boreham, R., Primatesta, P., Feyerabend, C., & Bryant, A. (2001). Nicotine yield from machine-smoked cigarettes and nicotine intakes in smokers: Evidence from a representative population survey. Journal of the National Cancer Institute, 93(2), 134-138. https://academic.oup.co

m/jnci/article/93/2/134/2906585

14. Janssen, I., Katzmarzyk, P. T., & Ross, R. (2004). Waist circumference and not body mass index explains obesity-related health risk. The American Journal of Clinical Nutrition, 79(3), 379-384. https://academic.oup.com/ajcn/article/79/3/379/4690123

15. Kennedy, D. O. (2016). B vitamins and the brain: Mechanisms, dose and efficacy—A review. Nutrients, 8(2), 68. https://www.mdpi.com/2072-6643/8/2/68

16. Kiecolt-Glaser, J. K., Gouin, J. P., & Hantsoo, L. (2010). Close relationships, inflammation, and health. Neuroscience & Biobehavioral Reviews, 35(1), 33-38. https://www.sciencedirect.com/science/article/abs/pii/S0149763410000155

17. Koob, G. F., & Colrain, I. M. (2012). Alcohol use disorder and sleep disturbances: A feed-forward allostatic framework. Neuropsychopharmacology, 37(1), 254-262. https://www.nature.com/articles/npp2011237

18. Kim, H.-G., Cheon, E.-J., Bai, D.-S., Lee, Y. H., & Koo, B.-H. (2018). Stress and heart rate variability: A meta-analysis and review of the literature. Psychiatry Investigation, 15(3), 235-245. https://www.ncbi.nlm.nih.gov/pmc/articles/PMC5606181/

19. Kupper, N. H., Willemsen, G., Posthuma, D., de Boer, D., Boomsma, D. I., & de Geus, E. J. (2005). A genetic analysis of ambulatory cardiorespiratory coupling. Psychophysiolo-

gy, 42(2), 202-212. https://onlinelibrary.wiley.com/doi/abs/10.1111/j.1469-8986.2005.00374.x

20. Laborde, S., Mosley, E., & Thayer, J. F. (2017). Heart rate variability and cardiac vagal tone in psychophysiological research–Recommendations for experiment planning, data analysis, and data reporting. Frontiers in Psychology, 8, 213. https://www.frontiersin.org/articles/10.3389/fpsyg.2017.00213/full

21. Lavie, C. J., De Schutter, A., & Milani, R. V. (2015). Healthy weight and obesity prevention: JACC health promotion series. Journal of the American College of Cardiology, 65(1), 1-2. https://www.jacc.org/doi/10.1016/j.jacc.2015.04.065

22. Lehrer, P., Vaschillo, E., Vaschillo, B., Lu, S. E., Scardella, A., Siddique, M., & Habib, R. (2004). Biofeedback treatment for asthma. Chest, 126(2), 352-361. https://journal.chestnet.org/article/S0012-3692(15)33791-6/fulltext

23. Libby, P. (2002). Inflammation in atherosclerosis. Nature, 420(6917), 868-874. https://www.nature.com/articles/420868a

24. Lief Blog. (n.d.). How to improve your HRV: 10 tips for better heart rate variability. Lief Therapeutics. Retrieved from https://blog.getlief.com/how-to-improve-your-hrv/

25. Lee, D., Seo, S. G., Lee, H., & Yoo, W. (2018). Effect of sitting posture on heart rate variability in young adults. Journal of Physical Therapy Science, 30(5), 661-664. https://www.ncbi.nlm.nih.gov/pmc/articles/PMC6088121/

26. Lehrer, P., & Gevirtz, R. (2014). Heart rate variability biofeedback: How and why does it work? Frontiers in Psychology, 5, 756. https://www.frontiersin.org/articles/10.3389/fpsyg.2014.00756/full

27. McCraty, R., & Shaffer, F. (2015). Heart rate variability: New perspectives on physiological mechanisms, assessment of self-regulatory capacity, and health risk. Global Advances in Health and Medicine, 4(1), 46-61. https://www.ncbi.nlm.nih.gov/pmc/articles/PMC4764425/

28. Michael, S., Graham, K. S., & Davis, G. M. (2017). Cardiac autonomic responses during exercise and post-exercise recovery using heart rate variability and systolic time intervals—A review. Frontiers in Physiology, 8, 301. https://www.frontiersin.org/articles/10.3389/fphys.2017.00301/full

29. Mozaffarian, D., & Wu, J. H. (2011). Omega-3 fatty acids and cardiovascular disease: Effects on risk factors, molecular pathways, and clinical events. Journal of the American College of Cardiology, 58(20), 2047-2067. https://www.jacc.org/doi/10.1016/j.jacc.2011.06.063

30. O'Sullivan, P. B., Grahamslaw, K. M., Kendell, M., Lapenskie, S. C., Möller, N. E., & Richards, K. V. (2002). The effect of different standing and sitting postures on trunk muscle activity in a pain-free population. Spine, 27(24), 1238-1244. https://journals.lww.com/spinejournal/Abstract/2002/10010/The_Effect_of_Different_Standing_and_Sitting.8.aspx

31. Plews, D. J., Laursen, P. B., Stanley, J., Kilding, A. E., &

Buchheit, M. (2013). Training adaptation and heart rate variability in elite endurance athletes: Opening the door to effective monitoring. Sports Medicine, 43(9), 773-785. https://link.springer.com/article/10.1007/s40279-013-0071-8

32. Popkin, B. M., D'Anci, K. E., & Rosenberg, I. H. (2010). Water, hydration, and health. Nutrition Reviews, 68(8), 439-458. https://academic.oup.com/nutritionreviews/article/68/8/439/1855872

33. Pressman, S. D., & Cohen, S. (2005). Does positive affect influence health? Psychological Bulletin, 131(6), 925-971. https://psycnet.apa.org/doi/10.1037/0033-2909.131.6.925

34. Purnell, J. Q., & Weyer, C. (2003). Cannabinoid receptors and the regulation of energy balance: A review of potential clinical implications. International Journal of Obesity, 27(3), 355-366. https://www.nature.com/articles/0802482

35. Quintana, D. S., & Heathers, J. A. J. (2014). Considerations in the assessment of heart rate variability in biobehavioral research. Frontiers in Psychology, 5, 805. https://www.frontiersin.org/articles/10.3389/fpsyg.2014.00805/full

36. Ranganathan, M., & D'Souza, D. C. (2006). The acute effects of cannabinoids on memory in humans: A review. Psychopharmacology, 188(4), 425-444. https://link.springer.com/article/10.1007/s00213-005-0178-0

37. Ristow, M., & Zarse, K. (2010). How increased oxidative stress promotes longevity and metabolic health: The concept of mitochondrial hormesis (mitohormesis). Experimental

Gerontology, 45(6), 410-418. https://www.sciencedirect.com/science/article/abs/pii/S0531556510001332

38. Russo, M. A., Santarelli, D. M., & O'Rourke, D. (2017). The physiological effects of slow breathing in the healthy human. Breathe, 13(4), 298-309. https://breathe.ersjournals.com/content/13/4/298

39. Sawka, M. N., Cheuvront, S. N., & Carter, R. (2005). Human water needs. Nutrition Reviews, 63(6), S30-S39. https://academic.oup.com/nutritionreviews/article/63/suppl_1/S30/1911892

40. Schroeder, E. B., Liao, D., Chambless, L. E., Prineas, R. J., Evans, G. W., Heiss, G., & Atherosclerosis Risk in Communities (ARIC) Study. (2003). Hypertension, blood pressure, and heart rate variability: The Atherosclerosis Risk in Communities (ARIC) study. Hypertension, 42(6), 1106-1111. https://www.ahajournals.org/doi/full/10.1161/01.HYP.0000100444.71069.73

41. Seals, D. R., & Esler, M. D. (2000). Human ageing and the sympathoadrenal system. Journal of Physiology, 528(3), 407-417. https://physoc.onlinelibrary.wiley.com/doi/full/10.1111/j.1469-7793.2000.t01-1-00671.x

42. Seppä, V. P., & Viik, J. (2019). A comparison of wrist-worn Polar and chest-worn Polar HR sensors for measuring heart rate variability. IEEE Journal of Biomedical and Health Informatics, 23(6), 2605-2612. https://ieeexplore.ieee.org/document/8646219

43. Singh, J. P., Larson, M. G., Tsuji, H., Evans, J. C., O'Donnell, C. J., & Levy, D. (1998). Reduced heart rate variability and new-onset hypertension: Insights into pathogenesis of hypertension: The Framingham Heart Study. Hypertension, 32(2), 293-297. https://www.ahajournals.org/doi/full/10.1161/01.HYP.32.2.293

44. Shaffer, F., & Ginsberg, J. P. (2017). An overview of heart rate variability metrics and norms. Frontiers in Public Health, 5, 258. https://www.frontiersin.org/articles/10.3389/fpubh.2017.00258/full

45. Shaffer, F., McCraty, R., & Zerr, C. L. (2014). A healthy heart is not a metronome: An integrative review of the heart's anatomy and heart rate variability. Frontiers in Psychology, 5, 1040. https://www.frontiersin.org/articles/10.3389/fpsyg.2014.01040/full

46. Temple, J. L., Bernard, C., Lipshultz, S. E., Czachor, J. D., Westphal, J. A., & Mestre, M. A. (2017). The safety of ingested caffeine: A comprehensive review. Frontiers in Psychiatry, 8, 80. https://www.frontiersin.org/articles/10.3389/fpsyt.2017.00080/full

47. Thayer, J. F., Åhs, F., Fredrikson, M., Sollers, J. J., & Wager, T. D. (2012). A meta-analysis of heart rate variability and neuroimaging studies: Implications for heart rate variability as a marker of stress and health. Neuroscience & Biobehavioral Reviews, 36(2), 747-756. https://www.sciencedirect.com/science/article/abs/pii/S0149763411001467

48. Thayer, J. F., & Lane, R. D. (2007). The role of vagal func-

tion in the risk for cardiovascular disease and mortality. Biological Psychology, 74(2), 224-242. https://www.sciencedirect.com/science/article/abs/pii/S0301051106002697

49. Thayer, J. F., Yamamoto, S. S., & Brosschot, J. F. (2010). The relationship of autonomic imbalance, heart rate variability, and cardiovascular disease risk factors. International Journal of Cardiology, 141(2), 122-131. https://www.sciencedirect.com/science/article/abs/pii/S0167527309008655

50. Uchino, B. N., Cacioppo, J. T., & Kiecolt-Glaser, J. K. (1996). The relationship between social support and physiological processes: A review with emphasis on underlying mechanisms and implications for health. Psychological Bulletin, 119(3), 488-531. https://psycnet.apa.org/doi/10.1037/0033-2909.119.3.488

51. Van Diest, I., Verstappen, K., Aubert, A. E., Widjaja, D., Vansteenwegen, D., & Vlemincx, E. (2014). Inhalation/exhalation ratio modulates the effect of slow breathing on heart rate variability and relaxation. Applied Psychophysiology and Biofeedback, 39(3-4), 171-180. https://link.springer.com/article/10.1007/s10484-014-9263-8

52. Vandrey, R., Smith, M. T., McCann, U. D., Budney, A. J., & Curran, E. M. (2011). Sleep disturbance and the effects of extended-release zolpidem during cannabis withdrawal. Sleep Medicine, 12(5), 487-494. https://www.sciencedirect.com/science/article/abs/pii/S1389945710004044

53. Vinik, A. I., Ziegler, D., & Diabetologia. (2007). Diabetic cardiovascular autonomic neuropathy. Diabetologia,

50(1), 67-78. https://link.springer.com/article/10.1007/s00125-006-0523-2

54. Walker, M. P. (2017). Why We Sleep: Unlocking the Power of Sleep and Dreams. Scribner.

55. Welltory. (n.d.). Heart rate variability: What it is and how you can harness its power. Welltory. Retrieved from https://welltory.com/heart-rate-variability/

56. Zeidan, F., Johnson, S. K., Diamond, B. J., David, Z., & Goolkasian, P. (2010). Mindfulness meditation improves cognition: Evidence of brief mental training. Consciousness and Cognition, 19(2), 597-605. https://www.sciencedirect.com/science/article/abs/pii/S1053810010001272

Printed in Dunstable, United Kingdom